The Low Sodium Cookbook

The Low Sodium Cookbook

DELICIOUS, SIMPLE, AND HEALTHY LOW-SALT RECIPES

SHASTA PRESS

Contents

Introduction

It is a surprising and comforting truth: reducing your sodium intake could save your life.

More than likely, you've picked up this book because your doctor has recommended that you adopt a low-sodium diet due to health issues. If you have been diagnosed with or are at high risk for developing high blood pressure, chronic kidney disease, osteoporosis, or a host of other diseases that can be caused or exacerbated by an excess of sodium in your system, your doctor is likely to recommend this type of diet. Or perhaps you are just hoping to optimize your health and avoid developing any of these troublesome conditions.

The most common diagnosis that leads to the recommendation of a low-sodium diet is hypertension, or high blood pressure, which can be lowered by reducing the amount of sodium in the diet. Reducing sodium intake can also help blood pressure medicines work better and prevent blood pressure from rising. Other diseases that have been connected to high sodium intake include ventricular hypertrophy and heart failure, osteoporosis, kidney stones and renal failure, edema, respiratory failure, gastric ulcers, and certain types of cancer. The good news is that even a small reduction in the amount of sodium in your diet can significantly improve your blood pressure and overall health.

If you've tried a low-sodium diet before, or even if this is the first time you've given it any thought at all, you might be thinking that you'll have to give up all the foods you love most, that this is a life sentence to live the rest of your days without delicious food. Happily, this book will prove that assumption wrong. In fact, many, maybe even most of your favorite foods can still be on your menu with a few recipe tweaks. The only foods that are really off-limits entirely are processed foods that contain excessive amounts of sodium and certain cured foods like bacon, salami, smoked fish, and the like.

Rest assured, though, that while you focus on reducing the amount of sodium in your diet, you'll enjoy a wide array of foods and a diet full of whole grains, fruits, vegetables, fresh meat, poultry, fish, seafood, low-fat dairy products, and even delectable sweets.

Changing your eating habits isn't easy, but this book will serve as a guide to small changes you can make in your habits to see big improvements. It will provide plenty of guidance on what to eat once you've eliminated the problem foods from your day-to-day menu.

Part I examines what sodium is and how it affects people's bodies and health, who should adopt a low-sodium diet, and what the health benefits of such a diet are. Guidelines will spell out what constitutes a low-sodium diet, offer tips for reducing sodium, and examine which foods are high in sodium and which are not.

A chapter on low-sodium eating will provide tips for shopping and cooking, reading food labels, and eating out without overdosing on salt. Finally, an outline detailing a two-week meal plan is included that will serve as a guide to get you started on your new way of eating.

Part II provides more than one hundred recipes for low-sodium dishes, including breakfasts, snacks, appetizers, condiments and sauces, soups, stews, salads, meat and poultry entrées, fish and seafood entrées, and tantalizing desserts. This book focuses on providing recipes for common favorite dishes and comfort foods to help you feel satisfied and fulfilled by your new diet, not deprived.

By reading this book, you'll learn:

- Simple tricks to easily reduce sodium in your diet

- How to recognize foods that contain "sneaky" or hidden sodium

- How to shop for low-sodium foods

- What foods contain health-enhancing vitamins, minerals, and other nutrients

- How to cook your favorite dishes with less sodium

Remember that even a small reduction in your sodium intake can have a significant effect on your health, and making small changes at every meal can add up to big results.

PART ONE

Understanding the Low-Sodium Diet

CHAPTER ONE

The Benefits of a Low-Sodium Diet

Why Choose a Low-Sodium Diet?

The simple answer is that you should choose a low-sodium diet because it could save your life.

The more complicated answer is that too much sodium in the diet can exacerbate certain conditions, especially high blood pressure, which puts undue pressure on your arteries, heart, kidneys, and other organs. It can make life uncomfortable, causing headaches, fatigue, shortness of breath, chest pain, and other unpleasant symptoms. And it also increases your risk of serious, even life-threatening illnesses, including diabetes, cancer, heart failure, respiratory failure, and osteoporosis.

When you have too much sodium in your system, it causes excess fluid to be held in the body, which puts added pressure on the circulatory system by increasing the force of blood against the artery walls. When this force is too strong, the pressure becomes burdensome to the heart and other organs. Therefore, consuming too much sodium increases your risk of cardiovascular diseases like hypertension, heart failure, and stroke. And this excessive pressure on the arterial walls can damage not just the heart but other organs and tissues, making you more susceptible to osteoporosis, stomach cancer, and kidney disease.

Chances are that you are embarking on a low-sodium diet not by choice but by necessity or because your doctor strongly advised that you cut your sodium intake to improve your health.

If you've been advised to adopt a low-sodium diet due to hypertension, you are not alone. Hypertension affects almost one out of every three people in the United States and is one of the leading causes of heart disease. Hypertension is often referred to as a "silent killer," because many sufferers aren't even aware that they have high blood pressure.

While sodium isn't the sole cause of high blood pressure—lack of exercise, obesity, and genetic factors are also culprits—cutting back on high-sodium foods is a simple way to significantly lower your risk of high blood pressure and its negative effects on the body.

What Is Sodium?

In its most basic form, sodium is a mineral that is found in nature, including in natural, unprocessed foods and in drinking water. Table salt is a compound of two minerals, sodium (40 percent) and chloride (60 percent). Sea salt, kosher salt, and other salts used to season food are also sodium chloride.

Much maligned as a dietary evil, sodium is actually one of the minerals most crucial for the healthy function of our bodies. It helps to regulate water balance, control muscle and nerve function, metabolize food, and keep our circulation running properly. Our bodies also need it to help regulate fluid levels and blood pressure. Ironically this last characteristic is where excess sodium in the diet often leads to problems when it causes our bodies to hang on to excess fluid, increasing the force of the blood on our artery walls and organs to dangerous levels. There is a fine balance between the right amount of sodium in our bodies and too much, which causes problems.

Many doctors recommend that patients who suffer from certain ailments, such as high blood pressure or edema—or are at high risk for developing such conditions—take pains to reduce the levels of sodium in their diets.

What Is a Low-Sodium Diet?

A low-sodium diet is one that limits the amount of sodium a person ingests, and it is often used to treat or prevent hypertension and other conditions.

The average American diet includes as much as 3,400 mg of sodium per day, which is twice the healthful level for most people. In fact, a sodium level no higher than 1,500 mg per day is recommended as a low-sodium diet.

Most of the sodium in our diet comes from table salt, or sodium chloride. Although sodium does occur naturally in unprocessed foods, the levels are low enough that these foods provide the quantities our bodies actually need, as opposed to the exorbitant levels found in many processed foods and even in home-cooked foods that incorporate large amounts of table salt.

There are two primary reasons that our diets have evolved to contain such high levels of sodium. The first is, of course, that salt is tasty and adds pleasant flavor to foods. This effect is intensified when salt is combined with fat and sugar, creating an even more dangerous combination. People's taste buds have become accustomed to saltier and saltier foods so that foods with little or no added salt, even if they contain naturally high levels of sodium, may taste bland.

The second reason sodium levels in our diets have skyrocketed is that salt is often used as an additive in processed foods, either to preserve or otherwise enhance them. It is added to many foods to inhibit the growth of food-borne pathogens and increase shelf life. It is also used to bind, stabilize, and enhance the color of many processed foods. This is why so many canned foods contain such extremely high levels of sodium, even when they don't taste particularly salty.

Reducing dietary sodium can be challenging since more than 75 percent of the sodium in a typical American's diet comes from processed or prepared foods, not salt used to season foods at the table or even during cooking. Becoming a savvy consumer and learning to scrutinize nutrition labels is the best way to identify the hidden sodium found in packaged foods.

There are even foods that don't come with labels, such as grains and meats, that are suspect. Their sodium levels might be low compared to highly processed foods, but their sodium content significantly contributes to our diets simply because people tend to eat so many servings of them in a day. A single slice of sandwich bread, for instance, may contain as much as 250 mg of sodium; a typical serving of dark-meat chicken may contain more than 450 mg of sodium.

With this in mind, it's easy to see how sodium quickly adds up, even if you eat a healthful diet of mostly homemade foods. And, of course, the problem is exacerbated the more you rely on prepared, highly processed, and fast foods.

It's good to remember that the main sources of sodium in our diets are:

- Certain condiments, such as soy sauce, steak sauce, and ketchup

- Cured meats, including cold cuts, bacon, and smoked fish

- Natural sources, including grains, vegetables, milk, cheese, meat, and shellfish

- Prepared foods, such as fast food and frozen meals

- Processed foods, such as canned soups, cereal, crackers, chips, bread, and jarred sauces

- Table salt, added to restaurant-prepared and home-cooked meals and at the table

On the most basic level, a low-sodium diet is one that includes less than 1,500 mg of sodium per day. This usually means strictly limiting processed foods and fast food and unnecessary added salt in recipes or at the table. It also means limiting some naturally high-sodium foods such as cheese, bacon, bread, cured meats and fish, and certain types of shellfish.

Who Should Follow a Low-Sodium Diet?

Low-sodium diets are most commonly recommended for people who suffer from or are at high risk of developing hypertension (high blood pressure) or heart disease, but anyone who suffers from hypertrophy, osteoporosis, kidney stones, renal failure, edema, shortness of breath, respiratory failure, gastric ulcers, or certain types of cancer is a prime candidate for a low-sodium diet.

If you have high or borderline high blood pressure, reducing your sodium intake can lower it. And if you are taking medication for high blood pressure, that's all the more reason you should adopt a low-sodium diet as it can enhance the effectiveness of the medication.

Some research has found that African Americans are more sensitive to sodium than others, which may be the reason that the African American population has a higher rate of high blood pressure. As a result, the Food and Drug Administration (FDA) includes African Americans of any age in the group of people who should limit sodium to 1,500 mg per day.

Even people with normal blood pressure can benefit from switching to a low-sodium diet, which will gradually lower their blood pressure, too, and decrease their risk of heart disease. And moderate sodium intake has been associated with numerous other health benefits, such as a reduced risk of dying from a stroke, reversal of heart enlargement, and a reduced risk of kidney stones and osteoporosis.

People with kidney problems should also limit their sodium intake. The kidneys help prevent sodium buildup in the body. Consuming more sodium than your kidneys can flush out can lead to swelling, spikes in blood pressure, breathing difficulties, and a buildup of fluid around the heart and lungs. Therefore, according to the National Kidney Foundation, if your kidneys are damaged or not functioning optimally, it's necessary to adopt a low-sodium diet.

The opposite but incredibly rare problem, sodium deficiency, can lead to a condition called hyponatremia, which may cause fatigue, seizures, muscle spasms, confusion, and coma. While following a low-sodium diet does slightly increase your risk of developing hyponatremia, it is extremely rare for a low-sodium diet to cause it. More often it is the result of certain medical conditions, vomiting, diarrhea, drinking excessive fluid (especially water), excessive sweating, or the use of certain medications.

Health Benefits of a Low-Sodium Diet

Following a low-sodium diet has many health benefits. First and foremost, of course, is reducing blood pressure, which in turn lowers the risk of heart attack and stroke.

While many hypertension sufferers don't even realize they have a problem until they go to the doctor, some people may experience bothersome symptoms such as severe headaches, fatigue, confusion, vision problems, chest pain, shortness of breath, or irregular heartbeat. All of these symptoms may be alleviated through a blood pressure–reducing low-sodium diet. In fact, when sodium intake is reduced, most people experience a drop in blood pressure within a few days to a few weeks.

An added benefit of a low-sodium diet is that it may help you drop unwanted pounds, which incidentally, can contribute to high blood pressure. If you currently eat more than the recommended daily maximum of sodium, it may be causing you to retain water, which can mean that you're carrying unnecessary weight. In fact, an excess of just 400 mg of sodium in your body can be responsible for an added two pounds of fluid. Drinking plenty of water can flush out excess sodium, causing those extra pounds to drop off, but unless you reduce your sodium intake, they will just pile right back on as the bloat returns.

In addition to raising blood pressure, sodium can cause your body to lose calcium, which weakens the bones over time and can lead to osteoporosis. Getting the recommended dose of calcium every day can help to offset the bone loss caused by a high-sodium diet, but reducing your salt intake goes right to the source, preventing a problem before it arises.

CHAPTER TWO

Low-Sodium Dietary Guidelines

How Much Sodium Is Too Much?

Opinions on the optimal level of sodium intake vary depending on who you ask, but the most reputable sources all agree on the minimum and maximum dietary levels of sodium for a healthful diet.

The average American consumes nearly 3,000 mg more of sodium each day that their body simply doesn't need. Our bodies actually need very little sodium to function optimally. A mere 500 mg of sodium is enough to keep our bodies running along smoothly. Therefore, reducing your sodium intake with a low-sodium diet has benefits no matter what your health condition.

Dietary Recommendations

As far as the upper limit of sodium in the diet, authoritative bodies such as the Institute of Medicine, the FDA, and the U.S. Department of Agriculture (USDA) all agree that even healthy adults should eat no more than 2,300 mg of sodium per day.

The Institute of Medicine considers 1,500 mg per day to be an "adequate intake level" and 2,300 mg per day to be the "tolerable upper intake level" for healthy adults between the ages of nineteen and fifty.

Healthy adults ages fifty to seventy; individuals of any age who suffer from hypertension, diabetes, or chronic kidney disease; or individuals of any age who are African American should consume no more than 1,500 mg. Individuals who are over the age of seventy, whose calorie requirements are lower than those of younger adults, should limit their sodium to 1,200 mg per day.

DAILY SODIUM LEVELS

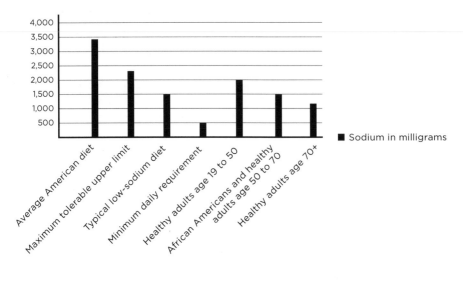

When this book refers to a low-sodium diet, it means a diet with a maximum 1,500 mg of sodium per day. If you are older than seventy, you should reduce the sodium in your diet by another 300 mg per day.

How Do I Follow a Low-Sodium Diet?

Following a low-sodium diet may seem daunting, especially if you are used to eating out often or frequently rely on frozen meals or other processed foods for meals at home, at the office, or elsewhere. Rest assured, though, that following a low-sodium diet is easy to do, and it doesn't mean that you have to give up all of your favorite foods. To the contrary, you may find that in your efforts to limit sodium, you'll discover new, fresh, homemade, nutritious foods that are even more delicious and satisfying than fast-food burgers, frozen pizza, or takeout burritos.

Remember that most of the sodium in our diets comes not from salt that is added at the table, or even during cooking, but from processed foods. These include chips, pretzels, and other snack foods; canned soups and broths; canned stews and chili; frozen meals; jarred pasta sauces and condiments; and pickles, olives, capers, and other foods packed in brine. Also included in this high-sodium category are breads, cured meats, and cheese.

Since more than 75 percent of the sodium in our diets comes from prepared, processed, and restaurant foods, that's a great place to start when looking to modify your diet. In a way, this is the easiest place to start, too, because the sodium content is listed right on the nutrition label of processed foods. Chain and fast-food restaurants are required to post nutritional information, including sodium content, on their menus. Many national restaurants also provide this information on their websites.

As you do your grocery shopping, get in the habit of reading labels. You may need to allow extra time to get your shopping done at first, but you'll gain valuable knowledge about the sodium content of the foods you eat. A good rule of thumb when you do choose processed foods is to stick to those that contain 140 mg of sodium or less per serving. This is the level that is considered to be low in sodium.

Once you start reading labels, you may find that many of the foods you eat regularly are now off the menu, but don't worry; you'll find plenty of delicious and healthful options to take their place.

Limiting your diet to mostly fresh, whole, and natural foods can take a big bite out of your daily sodium level. Fresh, whole foods without seasoning or sauces, such as fruits and vegetables—even those that naturally contain sodium—always fall within the low-sodium category. Choosing these foods whenever possible is a great start.

Canned foods, on the other hand, are almost always processed with a lot of sodium, unless they are marked "low sodium" or "no salt added." Of course, it's always better to choose fresh foods (or even frozen) over canned, but switching from high-sodium foods to these lower-sodium options will help you make significant cuts in your dietary sodium. Instead of canned beans, buy dried beans, for instance. The drawback is that these usually need to be soaked overnight and then cooked for an hour or two, but you'll cut the sodium by a ton.

Avoiding added salt, soy sauce, fish sauce, and other high-sodium sauces and condiments will go a long way toward reducing your sodium intake as well.

Cooking at home, from scratch, is the best way to make sure that you are sticking to your sodium limit, but restaurant dining and even fast foods aren't out of the question completely. When you do dine in a restaurant, check the nutritional information, choose carefully, and, whenever possible, ask for your meal to be prepared with minimal added salt or salty condiments.

Tell your family, loved ones, friends, and coworkers—anyone you share meals with on a regular basis—about your new low-sodium diet. This will help you garner support and make sure that others aren't inadvertently sabotaging your efforts when they cook for you. Who knows? You might even inspire others to join you in reducing sodium, or discover that someone you know is already on a low-sodium diet and might be able to share tips with you.

The goal is to keep your sodium intake to 1,500 mg or less per day. This means if you eat three meals and no snacks, you can have up to 500 mg per meal. However, be sure to count snacks, too. Many people like to limit the sodium of each meal to 350 mg and allow for two snacks per day with up to 225 mg of sodium.

When you embark on a low-sodium diet, it is extremely helpful to begin by tracking your sodium intake every day and at every meal. This is the best way to get a handle on how much sodium you're getting and where you might be able to easily cut back.

While you might prefer to use an old-fashioned pen-and-paper tracking method, there are lots of tracking apps available online—some are made to be used from your desktop or laptop and others can be used right on your smartphone or tablet. These programs do most of the work for you. All you have to do is enter in what you ate. At the end of the day, you'll be able to see exactly how much sodium you ate. This information can be quite valuable as you learn to make better choices.

Ten Tips for Reducing Sodium in Your Diet

1. Track your sodium intake every day and at every meal, at least until you become a savvy low-sodium dieter.

2. Choose fresh fruits and vegetables whenever possible. If fresh fruits and vegetables aren't available, opt for frozen over canned, and choose packages labeled "fresh frozen" that contain only the fruit or vegetable without added sauces or seasonings.

3. If canned fruits or vegetables are your only option, choose those labeled "low sodium" or "no salt added." Check the nutrition label as well.

4. When using canned foods (including fruits, vegetables, and beans), rinse the foods before using them. For canned tuna, buy no-salt-added varieties packed in water or oil.

5. Choose fresh, uncooked meats (steak, chicken, pork chops, etc.) over cured or processed meats (bacon, cooked ham, sausages, and deli meats like salami, pepperoni, or pastrami).

6. Steer clear of fermented or brined products (olives, sauerkraut, kimchi, capers, pickles, etc.) or use only very small quantities and rinse them well or soak them in water before using.

7. When cooking rice, pasta, beans, polenta, quinoa, couscous, or other starchy sides, omit the salt in the cooking water even if the package directions tell you to add it.

8. Limit the amount of cheese in your diet, and when you do eat cheese, look for lower-sodium versions.

9. Choose seasonings (spices, herbs, etc.) that do not contain any added salt or sodium. Garlic powder (not garlic salt), onion powder, cayenne or ground chipotle chilies and herbs like oregano, basil, rosemary, mint, and thyme add lots of flavor without boosting the sodium content of your meals.

10. Cook for yourself. Cooking at home, from scratch, using whole foods is the absolute best way to reduce the amount of sodium you consume.

CHAPTER THREE

High-and Low-Sodium Foods

Understanding Sodium Levels

As you get into the habit of researching the nutritional content of foods and reading nutritional labels, you'll soon develop a keen sense of which foods to avoid. As a general rule, the more highly processed a food is, the more sodium it is likely to contain. Whole foods, on the other hand, those that you consume more or less in the form in which you find them in nature, tend to be lower in sodium.

Of course, there are exceptions to every rule, and some whole, natural, unprocessed foods—like mussels, for example—are high in sodium. Do a bit of research so that you can avoid such unexpected sources of sodium.

Everyday Foods and Beverages High in Sodium

Everyone may point a finger at the salt shaker, but most of the salt people consume is hidden in prepared and processed foods. Many of the foods highest in sodium are the obvious culprits: the ready-to-eat foods people buy at the supermarket or pick up at a drive-through window on the way home from work. Some of them, however, may surprise you.

Bread has been called—by both the Centers for Disease Control and Prevention (CDC) and the American Heart Association—the number-one biggest saboteur of the low-sodium diet. One slice may contain as much as 250 mg of sodium. And even low-sodium breads can derail efforts to curb sodium intake simply because people tend to eat a lot of it.

It probably doesn't come as a big surprise that salami and ham are loaded with sodium, but even milder, "healthier" deli meats like roast turkey breast can deliver a shocking amount of sodium. In fact, a four-ounce serving of deli turkey may contain more than 1,000 mg of sodium, or two-thirds of your daily allotment. Put it between a couple of slices of bread and you're done for the day. Don't even think about adding cheese, mustard, or (gasp) pickles.

It may not be a big shocker that aged cheese—think salty blue cheese, sharp cheddar, and creamy Camembert—is high in sodium. But even mild cheeses that don't taste terribly salty, like cottage cheese, can have as much as 450 mg of sodium per serving.

Doing your research, comparing similar products, and choosing carefully are crucial to following a low-sodium diet. Take common types of cheese, for instance, which can vary dramatically in the amount of sodium they contain. Flavorful Swiss cheese contains a relatively low sodium level of 75 mg per ounce. Popular cheddar contains more than double that at 175 mg per ounce. And rich, salty blue cheese comes in at a whopping 400 mg per ounce.

Frozen meals are one of the most obvious culprits, with many delivering more than 800 mg per serving in their convenient heat-and-eat trays.

Canned soups, vegetables, and beans are more of the usual suspects, with some varieties containing as much as 900 mg per serving. Jarred spaghetti sauces, too, can top 550 mg per half-cup serving.

Condiments are sodium saboteurs, too. Compared to other foods, you may think that you consume so little of these sauces, marinades, and spreads that it's easy to dismiss them when you're adding up a meal's sodium content. But some of these tasty touches pack a shocking amount of sodium in just a spoonful. Mustard, which is relatively low in sodium for a condiment, contains more than 150 mg of sodium per tablespoon. Teriyaki sauce, on the other hand, contains nearly 700 mg of sodium per tablespoon, while the same amount of soy sauce contains 1,000 mg. And watch out, because even low-sodium soy sauce is likely to have more than 500 mg of sodium per tablespoon.

Don't be duped into thinking that prepared foods labeled "light," "lean," "low-fat," or "low-calorie" are likely to be lower in sodium. They're not. In fact, when manufacturers cut the fat and calories in foods, they often increase the salt to make up for any loss of flavor.

Here are a few common foods and beverages and their sodium content:

- 1 medium orange: 0 mg

- 1 medium apple: 2 mg

- ½ cup broccoli: 15 mg
- 1 (12-ounce) can of cola: 30 mg
- 1 cup mineral water: 40 mg
- 1 cup low-fat plain yogurt: 160 mg
- 1 tablespoon ketchup: 190 mg
- 4 saltine crackers: 280 mg
- ½ cup cottage cheese: 425 mg
- 1 hotdog: 560 mg
- 1 fast-food cheeseburger: 600 mg
- 1 slice pepperoni pizza: 680 mg
- 1 cup canned soup: 800 mg
- 1 tablespoon soy sauce: 1,000 mg
- 1 bean and cheese burrito: 1,030 mg
- 1 frozen beef enchilada meal: 1,800 mg

Which Foods Should I Eat and Which Foods Should I Avoid?

Let's start with the good news. There are plenty of nutritious, delicious, and low-sodium foods that you can and should eat to your heart's content. Foremost among them are fresh fruits and vegetables, eaten raw or steamed, sautéed, or roasted and seasoned with fresh herbs, sodium-free spices, lemon juice, vinegar, or other low-sodium ingredients.

Tomatoes are a good-for-you, low-sodium food, full of heart-healthful potassium and magnesium, plus hefty doses of beta-carotene and vitamin C, and only about 10 mg of sodium per cup. But make that a cup of canned tomato soup and the sodium level soars to 400 mg. Even worse, store-bought tomato juice registers more than 650 mg of sodium per cup. The worst offender? Store-bought tomato sauce, which delivers more than 1,000 mg of sodium per cup.

The number-one rule of low-sodium eating is to always choose food that is as close to the form in which it is found in nature as possible. For instance, fresh corn is better than frozen, frozen is better than canned, and canned corn kernels are better than canned corn chowder.

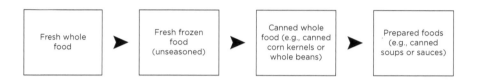

As a rule, try to eat fresh, unprocessed fruits and vegetables that you prepare yourself whenever you can. When fresh produce isn't an option, the next best choice is frozen produce that is fresh-frozen in its natural form with no seasonings or sauces added. Canned produce is a distant third, unless you can find low-sodium or no-salt-added versions. Canned soups, stews, and sauces and frozen or prepared meals should be avoided if at all possible, unless you can find versions that are truly low in sodium.

And remember, for every high-sodium food you have to give up, there is a flavorful and satisfying alternative just waiting for you to discover.

HIGH-SODIUM FOODS TO AVOID	LOW-SODIUM ALTERNATIVES
Smoked, cured, salted, or canned meat, including bacon, cold cuts, store-bought baked ham, hotdogs, and sausage	Fresh or frozen beef, lamb, pork, or other meat
Smoked or cured poultry, including smoked duck, chicken, and turkey	Fresh or frozen chicken, turkey, duck, or other poultry
Salty preserved or canned fish, including sardines, caviar, and anchovies	Fresh or frozen fish, low-sodium canned fish, and water- or oil-packed canned tuna
Fresh or frozen mussels and canned or smoked clams, mussels, or oysters	Fresh or frozen shrimp, lobster, crab, clams, and oysters
Olives, pickles, capers, sauerkraut, kimchi, other pickled or fermented vegetables, and canned chilies	Fresh chilies, fresh shredded cabbage or other vegetables, and minced onions
Frozen dinners, such as burritos and pizza	Home-cooked meals or low-sodium meals (less than 140 mg of sodium per serving)

HIGH-SODIUM FOODS TO AVOID	LOW-SODIUM ALTERNATIVES
Canned prepared foods, such as ravioli, soup, and chili	Homemade foods, fresh or dried pasta cooked without salt, and canned low-sodium soups (less than 140 mg of sodium per serving)
Canned beans	Dried beans, soaked and cooked without added salt
Canned vegetables	Fresh or fresh-frozen vegetables
Regular and processed cheese, cheese spreads, cheese sauce, and cottage cheese	Low-sodium cheeses, ricotta cheese, and part-skim mozzarella cheese
Bread and rolls with salt on top	Bread and rolls without salt on top
Quick breads, self-rising flour, and biscuit, pancake, and waffle mixes	Muffins and many ready-to-eat cereals
Prepackaged, processed mixes for potatoes, rice, pasta, and stuffing	Rice, pasta, and potatoes cooked without added salt
Store-bought pasta sauce, tomato sauce, and salsa	Homemade sauces and salsas without added salt or store-bought low-sodium versions (less than 140 mg of sodium per serving)
Salted chips, pretzels, crackers, popcorn, and salted nuts	Unsalted chips, pretzels, crackers, popcorn, nuts, and fresh vegetable crudités
Soy sauce and fish sauce	Vinegar and citrus juice
Ketchup and mustard	Mayonnaise, vinegar, and citrus juice
Salted butter and margarine	Unsalted butter and margarine
Bottled salad dressings	Homemade dressings without added salt, or store-bought low-sodium versions
Peanut butter and other nut or seed butters (almond, cashew, sunflower seed)	All-natural peanut butter and other nut or seed butters with no salt added, and tahini (sesame seed paste)
Instant pudding and cake mixes	Ice cream and frozen yogurt

Sneaky Sodium

By now you're probably pretty savvy about recognizing obvious high-sodium foods like salted nuts, chips, and cheeseburgers, but there's a whole range of foods that stealthily deliver sodium bombs without us even realizing it. To spot them, you have to be vigilant about reading labels and comparing brands.

Many grain-based foods like breads, rolls, and tortillas fall into this sneaky category. A large regular flour tortilla might contain 450 mg of sodium. A regular corn tortilla, on the other hand, can come in with a sodium level as low as 10 mg.

Likewise, instant rice contains as much as 600 mg of sodium per cup, while regular rice cooked without added salt contains almost none (2 mg per cup). Rice cooked with seasonings, such as yellow rice, Spanish rice, or rice pilaf, may top 1,000 mg of sodium per cup.

As previously discussed, condiments are often high in sodium, especially when you consider how much of them you might eat in a sitting. Now let's look at those little flavor packets that come in boxed rice mixes, noodle soup mixes, or other just-add-water foods. Take ramen soup mix, as an example. That tiny, innocent-looking flavor packet often contains 900 mg of sodium. And the packet that comes in boxed rice mixes often tops 600 mg of sodium per serving.

The breakfast cereal aisle is another minefield for anyone trying to avoid excess sodium. Even the "healthful," all-natural, no-sugar-added varieties of breakfast cereal are often loaded with sodium. One popular brand of raisin bran contains 280 mg of sodium per serving. And who among us hasn't gobbled two (or more!) servings while reading the morning paper?

And then there's the beverage aisle, which might seem like the safest place of all, but even here you have to check labels. For instance, you might be tempted to grab a vegetable juice to sneak in a serving or two of healthful vegetables without really trying, but you'd likely be sneaking in a whopping 480 mg of sodium per serving. Sports drinks, which are designed to replenish sodium that has been lost through sweat, are also, as you'd expect, high in sodium. And even low-fat milk has 100 mg of sodium per cup.

The bottom line is, until this new low-sodium diet becomes second nature for you, you're going to have to read labels, compare and contrast, research, research, research, and track your sodium intake.

Naturally Low-Sodium Foods

As mentioned previously, there are many delicious, nutritious, and satisfying foods that are naturally low in sodium. Among these are fruits and vegetables (fresh, or frozen without added seasonings); fruits; meats, poultry, and fish (fresh, or frozen without added seasonings); whole grains such as rice, wheat, oats, quinoa, and barley; fresh and dried herbs; spices (excluding spice mixes that contain salt); and flavorful ingredients like citrus juice, vinegar, and unsalted butter.

Alternative Seasonings

The primary use of salt in home cooking, of course, is to add flavor. And no one wants to be sentenced to a diet of bland foods for the rest of their life. Not to worry; there are a million and one ways to spice up your meals without adding even a grain of salt.

Fresh and dried herbs and spices can add complex layers of flavor. From basil, oregano, and thyme to turmeric, smoked paprika, cayenne, or dried mustard, there are many ways to flavor savory dishes with herbs and spices. When using spice mixes, like curry powder, just be sure to check the label for added salt.

There are also herbs and spices that complement sweet dishes as well as savory ones. Ginger, cinnamon, allspice, cloves, nutmeg, and mint are just a few such multi-purpose seasonings.

Of course, aromatic vegetables are another source of intense flavors. Onions, garlic, shallots, chilies, and leeks complement meat, fish, or vegetable dishes. Onion powder and garlic powder, too, are a convenient way to add flavor to dishes (just don't confuse garlic powder with garlic salt).

Vinegars offer tons of seasoning variety, too. To start, there are vinegars made from red wine, white wine, champagne, and sherry. There are fruity vinegars like apple cider, raspberry, or fig. And vinegars come infused with herbs, too, such as tarragon or thyme.

And let's not forget oils. Ubiquitous olive oil adds fruity and earthy flavor all by itself. Then there are oils infused with fruits, herbs, and spices: Meyer lemon, rosemary, roasted garlic, and other intensely flavored oils pump up the flavor profile of a dish with just a drizzle, and without adding any sodium. And last, but by no means least, toasted sesame oil and chili oil flavor many favorite Asian dishes.

Citrus fruits are another great low-sodium source of flavor. Both the juice and the zest of lemons, limes, oranges, grapefruits, and even kumquats can be used to flavor everything from salad dressings to desserts.

Low-Sodium Substitutes

Several manufacturers make salt substitutes that are designed to both replace salt in cooking and substitute it for seasoning food at the table. These salt substitutes are made primarily of potassium chloride, which is a sodium-free salt (it is made up of potassium and chloride instead of sodium and chloride like table salt). While these substitutes don't taste or function exactly like salt, they can be used to add a "saltiness" to foods without the sodium.

Check with your doctor before using salt substitutes. The FDA has warned that although these substitutes are safe for healthy folks, they could be dangerous for people who have kidney disease, diabetes, or heart disease, or who take certain medications.

As more and more people adopt low-sodium diets, food manufacturers are responding with versions of their products with reduced sodium levels. According to the FDA, in order to be labeled "low sodium," a food must contain less than 140 mg of sodium per serving. When purchasing prepared foods, look for these low-sodium versions, but don't forget to watch your portion size. What you think of as a serving may not be the same as what's indicated on the label.

Many canned vegetables and fruits these days can also be found labeled "no salt added." Remember, this means that no additional salt has been added to the product during cooking or processing, but it doesn't mean that it is sodium-free. You should still check the label and include the sodium content in your tracking.

CHAPTER FOUR

Low-Sodium Eating

The Low-Sodium Diet Challenge

Talking about a low-sodium diet is all well and good in theory, but actually eating low-sodium food all day, every day is the real challenge. As previously discussed, there are plenty of low-sodium alternatives for your favorite foods, but incorporating them into your diet, and more important, nixing the high-sodium versions, can be difficult.

Remember to drink eight (or more!) glasses of water a day. Water flushes sodium from your body, which is an important part of reducing blood pressure. Get in the habit of keeping a glass or bottle of water nearby and sipping throughout the day.

Making a change in your diet as drastic as reducing your daily sodium intake from, say, 3,000 mg to the recommended 1,500 mg isn't easy, but here are the essentials boiled down to five easy-to-remember steps:

1. Stop adding salt to your food, either while cooking or at the table (this includes condiments like soy sauce).

2. Limit prepared foods and fast foods to once-in-a-while treats or emergency conveniences. When you do opt for these foods, choose low-sodium versions.

3. Get in the habit of reading nutritional information labels and choose foods that are naturally low in sodium.

4. Become acquainted (or reacquainted, as the case may be) with your kitchen and spice cabinet. Cook most of your meals at home so that you can control what does and doesn't get added.

5. Choose whole, natural foods over processed foods whenever possible.

Eventually, your body will adjust to your new diet and you'll stop missing the added salt. In fact, you may be surprised to find that within a couple of months you will be so used to low-sodium eating that foods you used to enjoy, like potato chips or French fries, taste much too salty to you now.

Cooking Tips and Techniques

Frequently eating prepared foods or eating out makes following a low-sodium diet especially challenging. The best—and dare we say, the easiest—way to reduce the sodium in your diet is to cook most of your food yourself. This way, you know exactly what goes into it and you can make adjustments, like adding additional spices to make up for a lack of salt, to ensure that the food will be delicious.

Seek out low-sodium recipes for your favorite foods, or adapt recipes yourself. The second half of this book provides more than one hundred recipes for favorite foods—from refreshing salads to spicy chilies, hearty grilled steak and beef stew to light grilled-fish dishes, as well as virtuous fruit desserts and luscious, but still low-fat, chocolate cream pie.

The more you cook low-sodium dishes, the more adept you'll become at using low-sodium substitutes. Soon it will become second nature. And once you've mastered low-sodium cooking, almost no meal will be off-limits to you. Whether it's pizza, tuna casserole, or spaghetti and meatballs you crave, you can adapt recipes to fit your low-sodium requirements.

The first rule of low-sodium cooking, just like low-sodium eating, is to choose whole, natural, fresh ingredients over processed foods whenever possible. Start with fresh tomatoes instead of canned, if you can, and you'll immediately cut a huge amount of sodium. Dried beans are another place where starting from scratch can drastically reduce the sodium content, so start with dried beans instead of canned. Soak and cook a large batch and store them in can-size portions in your freezer to make substituting them for canned in recipes a cinch. Cooked beans will keep in your freezer for up to three months.

The same goes for chicken, beef, or vegetable broths. Make your own from scratch, and not only will you know exactly what is in it, but you can control the salt and other seasonings to ensure that your broth is flavorful without being loaded with sodium. And again, you can make large batches and freeze them in can-size portions for easy substituting. If you don't have time to make your own broth, by all means, choose a low-sodium version or dilute it with water.

And, of course, don't add salt to the food you are cooking. Many foods naturally contain sodium, and condiments often do, too, so adding table salt is unnecessary. But remember, low-sodium doesn't have to mean bland. Take some time to explore the spice aisle at your supermarket and you'll find dozens of ways to spice up your meals. Even if a recipe calls for just a pinch of salt, find another seasoning to replace it.

Even when the cooking directions on the package say to add salt, don't! It's common for the directions for cooking dried pasta, rice, and other grains or grain-based foods to instruct you to add salt, but rest assured, this isn't necessary. The food will cook up just fine without it, and you don't need the extra sodium.

Spices like ground dried chilies, peppercorns, cumin, fennel seeds, cinnamon, and ground mustard can be combined in a million different ways to create varied flavor profiles. Dried herbs, too, are a convenient way to bring various dishes to life. Basil or oregano make your spaghetti sauce taste like authentic Italian cooking. Curry powder makes it easy to reproduce some of your favorite Indian restaurant's dishes at home. Ground chipotle powder is perfect for spicing up meat for tacos.

In the produce section, you'll find fresh herbs like cilantro, oregano, rosemary, thyme, sage, mint, and parsley that can add even more vibrant flavor to your dishes. Stirring a handful of chopped fresh herbs into a soup or stew at the last minute really brings the flavors to life.

And while you're in the produce aisle, be sure to pick up some lemons, limes, garlic, fresh ginger, onions, shallots, green onions, and leeks. All of these commonly available ingredients are low in sodium and add tons of flavor to any dish.

Some foods like pickles, olives, and capers can be used only in very small amounts. A tablespoon of capers in a dish that serves eight is fine, but a tablespoon of capers on your bagel with cream cheese is not. When you do use these ingredients in your cooking, use the most flavorful brands or varieties you can find and use them sparingly.

Regular soy sauce is sadly one ingredient that really has no place in a low-sodium household since even just one teaspoon contains nearly a quarter of an entire day's sodium allotment. Other condiments like Worcestershire sauce, mustard, and ketchup should be replaced with low-sodium or no-salt-added varieties or used only in small amounts.

Here are a few simple ideas for adding flavor to your meals without adding sodium:

- Use an acidic fruit juice—lemon, lime, orange, or even pineapple—along with some fresh or dried herbs or ground spices as a marinade for meat, poultry, or fish.

- Coat fish or chicken with sesame seeds before pan-searing.

- Add sautéed onions, shallots, leeks, or garlic to sautéed, stir-fried, or braised dishes.

- Add dried fruits—apricots, cranberries, raisins, or figs—to salads, grains, or even meat stews for extra zing.

- Season steamed vegetables with a drizzle of toasted sesame oil and/or a sprinkling of toasted sesame seeds.

- Spice up dishes with a drizzle of chili oil or a sprinkling of cayenne.

- Toss diced potatoes with olive oil and minced fresh rosemary and then roast them in a hot oven until crisp on the outside and tender inside.

- Season corn on the cob with fresh-squeezed lime juice and (salt-free) chili powder.

- Toss hot pasta with olive oil, minced fresh garlic, and thinly sliced fresh basil.

Learn to Read Food Labels

Reading food labels is an important part of making the switch to a low-sodium diet. There is so much hidden sodium in packaged foods that the only way you can know how much you are getting and what foods to avoid is to read every single label.

First, check the serving size and think about how much of that food you normally eat. Ketchup, for instance, has a serving size of one tablespoon, but most people eat three or four times that (at least) with a basket of French fries.

Next, check the sodium content and multiply that number by how many servings you're likely to eat in a meal. Using ketchup as an example, if you think you'll eat three tablespoons, and the sodium per serving listed on the package is 200 mg, then 600 mg is the amount of sodium you'd likely consume in a meal that includes that particular ketchup.

When buying canned or packaged foods, look for labels that read "reduced sodium," "low sodium," or "no salt added." Choose the no-salt or low-sodium options whenever possible. Remember, "low sodium" means that the food contains less than 140 mg of sodium per serving, and "no salt added" means that no salt is added during the cooking or processing, even though the food in the package might naturally contain some sodium.

Ten Tips for Dining Out

The toughest thing about eating out when you are on a low-sodium diet is figuring out just how much sodium you are getting since you don't know how the foods are prepared or exactly what is being added. Still, it is possible to eat out without sending your low-sodium diet off the rails. Here are ten tips to help you navigate a low-sodium diet in a restaurant setting:

1. Steer clear of fast-food and chain restaurants where the workers have little control over the individual ingredients in your meal. If you can't avoid going to a fast-food restaurant, check the nutrition information, which should be posted in the restaurant (and might be available on the restaurant's website) to find the lowest-sodium options. Ask for high-sodium condiments like ketchup, mustard, or salad dressing to be left off or served on the side.

2. When possible, choose individually owned (nonchain) restaurants where food is cooked to order.

3. Ask your server questions about how the food is prepared and what goes into the dish. If he doesn't know, ask him to check with the chef.

4. Speak up. Don't be shy about telling your server that you are on a strict low-sodium diet and asking for your food to be prepared without added salt or high-sodium condiments if at all possible.

5. Go for something simple, like grilled or roasted meat or fish, rather than a complicated curry, braised dish, or casserole that has many ingredients. The more ingredients a dish has, the more likely some of them are high in sodium.

6. Ask for the sauce to be left off your dish or served on the side.

7. Use condiments sparingly, if at all. Remember, condiments often contain more hidden sodium than you might expect.

8. Don't add additional salt to your food at the table. If you are tempted, ask the server to remove the salt shaker. Better yet, pack your own salt-free spice mixture and stash it in your purse or pocket to add to anything that is too bland for your taste.

9. Skip salty accoutrements like olives, pickles, capers, or grated cheese.

10. Enjoy a fruit-based dessert.

CHAPTER FIVE

14-Day Low-Sodium Meal Plan

Low-Sodium Action Plan

Starting any new lifestyle habit—whether it is an exercise plan or a diet—is challenging since habits are deeply ingrained and often hard to break or even bend. Having a detailed plan is a great way to get you started on the right track. It's like a road map that shows you exactly where to turn every step of the way.

Our fourteen-day meal plan is designed to help get you off on the right foot by providing a detailed guideline for you to follow for the first two weeks of your low-sodium diet. The 14-Day Low-Sodium Meal Plan is designed for the typical adult with a maximum of 1,500 mg of sodium per day. You may need to make adjustments to suit your own particular requirements. (See the dietary recommendations in Chapter 2, page 8, for more information.)

Remember that your low-sodium diet is a lifestyle change, not a quick fix. You may find that after just a few weeks on the diet, your blood pressure drops significantly and troublesome symptoms begin to disappear. Don't fall into the trap of thinking that you've fixed the problem and can go back to your old habits. Returning to a high-sodium diet will ensure only that all of those problems will come back to haunt you again. The key is to start and stay on a low-sodium diet.

The good news is that once you've been on the diet for a few weeks, you'll find that choosing low-sodium foods becomes second nature. You won't have to think so much about every morsel of food that you put in your mouth. Soon you will be eating a low-sodium diet as a matter of course, with hardly a second thought.

All of the foods on this plan are familiar and easy to find in your regular supermarket or grocery store. Remember to always drink water with your meals and throughout the day to keep your system clean and moving. Included in the fourteen-day meal plan are many of the recipes from this book. The recipes, of course, are all easy to make, full of flavor, and low in sodium.

Note: the recipes from this book are marked with a star (*) in the meal plan.

Day 1 (total sodium 1,241 mg)

BREAKFAST (215 MG SODIUM)

1 toasted whole-wheat English muffin with
- 2 tablespoons no-salt-added all-natural peanut butter and
- 1 teaspoon honey (106 mg sodium)

1 medium apple (2 mg sodium)
1 cup 1 percent low-fat milk (107 mg sodium)

MID-MORNING SNACK (145 MG SODIUM)

1 medium peach
1 cup low-fat fruit-flavored yogurt (145 mg sodium)

LUNCH (475 MG SODIUM)

Heart-Healthful Cobb Salad* (390 mg sodium) with
- 2 tablespoons low-sodium croutons (85 mg sodium)

MID-AFTERNOON SNACK (194 MG SODIUM)

14 whole-grain low-sodium crackers (170 mg sodium)
Jalapeño-Cilantro Hummus* (24 mg sodium)

DINNER (162 MG SODIUM)

1 (4-ounce) halibut fillet coated with 1 tablespoon crushed pecans and
¼ teaspoon freshly ground pepper, pan-fried in ½ tablespoon unsalted butter
(120 mg sodium)
½ cup cooked quinoa tossed with ½ cup chopped fresh tomato, ½ cup diced
cucumber, and 1 teaspoon fresh lemon juice (12 mg sodium)
1 cup steamed broccoli (30 mg sodium)

DESSERT (50 MG SODIUM)

½ cup chocolate ice cream topped with
- ½ cup sliced strawberries (50 mg sodium)

Day 2 (1,367 mg sodium)

BREAKFAST (208 MG SODIUM)

1 Healthful Apple Muffin with Cinnamon-Pecan Topping* (136 mg sodium)
1 hard-boiled egg (70 mg sodium)
1 cup fresh orange juice (2 mg sodium)

MID-MORNING SNACK (150 MG SODIUM)

1 (1-ounce) slice low-sodium Muenster cheese (75 mg sodium)
20 unsalted mini pretzels (75 mg sodium)

LUNCH (497 MG SODIUM)

Tuna salad sandwich
- 2 slices 100 percent whole-wheat sandwich bread (292 mg sodium)
- 3 ounces light, water-packed tuna (no salt added) mixed with 1 tablespoon minced celery, 2 teaspoons minced red onion, 1 tablespoon light mayonnaise, and 1 teaspoon fresh lemon juice (154 mg sodium)
- 1 large lettuce leaf (5 mg sodium)
- 2 slices tomato (1 mg sodium)
½ cup carrot sticks (45 mg sodium)

MID-AFTERNOON SNACK (3 MG SODIUM)

1 medium pear (2 mg sodium)
15 unsalted almonds (1 mg sodium)

DINNER (489 MG SODIUM)

Pan-Roasted Chicken Breast in Dijon Sauce* (459 mg sodium)
Green salad with 2 tablespoons low-fat vinaigrette (20 mg sodium)
1 cup potatoes roasted with 1 teaspoon olive oil, ¼ teaspoon freshly ground pepper, and ¼ teaspoon freshly minced rosemary (10 mg sodium)

DESSERT (20 MG SODIUM)

1 cup fresh berries with
- ½ cup frozen all-natural whipped topping (20 mg sodium)

Day 3 (1,139 mg sodium)

BREAKFAST (298 MG SODIUM)

1¼ cup toasted rice cereal (190 mg sodium) with
- 1 cup 1 percent low-fat milk (107 mg sodium)
- ½ cup fresh blueberries (1 mg sodium)

MID-MORNING SNACK (4 MG SODIUM)

1 medium banana (1 mg sodium)
1 tablespoon no-salt-added all-natural peanut butter (3 mg sodium)

LUNCH (461 MG SODIUM)

Smoky Red Lentil Soup* (153 mg sodium) with
- ½ cup cooked quinoa mixed in (6 mg sodium)
1 (3-inch) piece whole-wheat baguette (300 mg sodium)
1 medium apple (2 mg sodium)

MID-AFTERNOON SNACK (55 MG SODIUM)

1 cup snap peas (5 mg sodium)
¼ cup Fresh Garlic and Herb Yogurt Dip* (50 mg sodium)

DINNER (250 MG SODIUM)

Seared Salmon with Cilantro-Lime Pesto* (205 mg sodium)
1 cup steamed snow peas (6 mg sodium)
1 medium baked sweet potato (40 mg sodium)

DESSERT (71 MG SODIUM)

½ cup low-fat vanilla frozen yogurt (70 mg sodium)
½ cup sliced strawberries (1 mg sodium)

Day 4 (1,444 mg sodium)

BREAKFAST (350 MG SODIUM)

Speedy breakfast taco
- 2 corn tortillas
- 2 scrambled eggs (scrambled in a nonstick pan coated with cooking spray) (182 mg sodium)
- 2 tablespoons shredded reduced-fat cheddar cheese (64 mg sodium)
- 2 tablespoons tomato salsa (150 mg sodium)

1 cup fresh orange juice (2 mg sodium)

MID-MORNING SNACK (173 MG SODIUM)

1 medium apple (2 mg sodium)
1 (1-ounce) slice low-fat cheddar cheese (171 mg sodium)

LUNCH (424 MG SODIUM)

Spinach salad with shrimp
- 2 ounces cooked shrimp (342 mg sodium)
- 3 cups baby spinach (72 mg sodium)
- 1 small ripe avocado, peeled, pitted, and sliced (7 mg sodium)
- ½ cup halved cherry tomatoes (3 mg sodium)
- 1 tablespoon fresh lemon juice mixed with 2 teaspoons olive oil
- 2 tablespoons toasted pine nuts

MID-AFTERNOON SNACK (159 MG SODIUM)

Curry-Lime Peanuts* (155 mg sodium)
1 ounce seedless raisins (4 mg sodium)

DINNER (308 MG SODIUM)

Pork Chops with Green Peppercorn Sauce* (290 mg sodium)
1 baked potato with 1 tablespoon unsalted butter (17 mg sodium)
1 cup steamed green beans (1 mg sodium)

DESSERT (30 MG SODIUM)

½ cup raspberry sorbet (15 mg sodium) with
- 2 tablespoons chocolate syrup (15 mg sodium)

Day 5 (1,140 mg sodium)

BREAKFAST (25 MG SODIUM)

Rise and Shine Fruit Smoothie* (25 mg sodium)

MID-MORNING SNACK (149 MG SODIUM)

1 slice whole-wheat toast with
- 1 tablespoon no-salt-added all-natural peanut butter (149 mg sodium)

LUNCH (424 MG SODIUM)

Quick chicken tacos
- 2 small corn tortillas (6 mg sodium)
- 4 ounces cooked boneless skinless chicken breast, shredded (10 mg sodium)
- ½ cup canned black beans, drained and rinsed (166 mg sodium)
- ½ small ripe avocado, peeled, pitted, and sliced (3 mg sodium)
- ¼ cup fresh salsa (229 mg sodium)
- ½ cup shredded cabbage (8 mg sodium)

1 medium apple (2 mg sodium)

MID-AFTERNOON SNACK (114 MG SODIUM)

6 ounces low-fat peach yogurt with 2 tablespoons granola (114 mg sodium)

DINNER (351 MG SODIUM)

Seared Trout with Cherry Tomatoes and Bacon* (338 mg sodium)
1 cup cooked quinoa (13 mg sodium)
1 cup roasted zucchini cooked with olive oil spray and freshly ground pepper (8 mg sodium)

DESSERT (77 MG SODIUM)

2 ounces part-skim ricotta cheese with
- 3 sliced figs
- 2 teaspoons honey
- 1 tablespoon chopped pistachios (77 mg sodium)

Day 6 (1,134 mg sodium)

BREAKFAST (213 MG SODIUM)

1 whole-wheat English muffin with
- 2 tablespoons no-salt-added all-natural peanut butter
- ½ sliced banana (106 mg sodium)

1 cup 1 percent low-fat milk (107 mg sodium)

MID-MORNING SNACK (170 MG SODIUM)

1 cup diced melon
2 graham crackers (170 mg sodium)

LUNCH (398 MG SODIUM)

Baby Blues Salad* (298 mg sodium)
3 ounces cooked chicken breast, skin removed (98 mg sodium)
1 medium pear (2 mg sodium)

MID-AFTERNOON SNACK (105 MG SODIUM)

Lemon-Pepper Popcorn with Parmesan* (105 mg sodium)

DINNER (238 MG SODIUM)

6 ounces pan-seared tilapia cooked in 1 tablespoon unsalted butter, topped with
- ¼ cup mango or papaya salsa (155 mg sodium)

6 ounces baked sweet potato fries cooked with olive oil spray and freshly ground pepper (60 mg sodium)
1 cup Brussels sprouts roasted with ¼ small, diced onion and olive oil spray (23 mg sodium)

DESSERT (10 MG SODIUM)

1½ ounces dark chocolate (10 mg sodium)

Day 7 (1,181 mg sodium)

BREAKFAST (135 MG SODIUM)

Maple-Cinnamon Oatmeal Pancakes* (130 mg sodium) with
- 2 tablespoons maple syrup (2 mg sodium)
- 1 cup fresh berries (1 mg sodium)

1 cup fresh orange juice (2 mg sodium)

MID-MORNING SNACK (200 MG SODIUM)

1 medium peach
1 (1-ounce) slice low-fat cheddar cheese (171 mg sodium)
1 brown rice cake (29 mg sodium)

LUNCH (339 MG SODIUM)

Open-faced turkey sandwich
- 1 slice whole-wheat bread (146 mg sodium)
- 2 ounces low-sodium sliced turkey breast (84 mg sodium)
- 1 teaspoon Dijon mustard (57 mg sodium)
- 1 teaspoon light mayonnaise (34 mg sodium)
- ½ small avocado, peeled, pitted, and mashed (3 mg sodium)
- 2 slices tomato (1 mg sodium)
- 1 lettuce leaf (5 mg sodium)

1 cup sugar snap peas (6 mg sodium)
1 small bunch grapes (3 mg sodium)

MID-AFTERNOON SNACK (106 MG SODIUM)

1 red bell pepper, cut into strips (6 mg sodium)
Roasted Garlic and Rosemary Spread* (100 mg sodium)

DINNER (381 MG SODIUM)

4 ounces grilled flank steak marinated in lime juice, olive oil, fresh oregano, garlic, cumin, and chili powder (64 mg sodium)
6 ounces Swiss chard sautéed in olive oil spray with 1 minced garlic clove (304 mg sodium)
1 cup cooked quinoa (13 mg sodium)

DESSERT (20 MG SODIUM)

1 chocolate-dipped frozen banana (20 mg sodium)

Day 8 (1,264 mg sodium)

BREAKFAST (188 MG SODIUM)

Cherry-Almond Granola* (81 mg sodium) with
- 1 cup 1 percent low-fat milk (107 mg sodium)

MID-MORNING SNACK (170 MG SODIUM)

½ cup unsweetened applesauce (10 mg sodium)
2 graham crackers (160 mg sodium)

LUNCH (442 MG SODIUM)

Green salad with tuna, apples, and pecans
- 2 cups chopped romaine lettuce (20 mg sodium)
- 3 ounces white tuna packed in water (320 mg sodium)
- ½ medium apple, cored and diced (1 mg sodium)
- 2 tablespoons chopped pecans
- ¼ red onion, thinly sliced (3 mg sodium)
- Garlic-Dijon Vinaigrette* (98 mg sodium)

MID-AFTERNOON SNACK (154 MG SODIUM)

1 ounce unsalted baked tortilla chips (4 mg sodium) with
- 2 tablespoons fresh salsa (150 to 229 mg sodium)

DINNER (240 MG SODIUM)

Moroccan-Spiced Lamb Tagine* (226 mg sodium)
1 cup couscous (8 mg sodium)
Salad of diced cucumber, tomato, and red onion, with fresh lemon juice and parsley
(6 mg sodium)

DESSERT (70 MG SODIUM)

Vanilla low-fat frozen yogurt with fresh berries (70 mg sodium)

Day 9 (1,458 mg sodium)

BREAKFAST (344 MG SODIUM)

½ whole-wheat bagel (270 mg sodium) with
- 1 tablespoon light cream cheese (70 mg sodium)

1 cup fresh orange juice (2 mg sodium)

1 medium apple (2 mg sodium)

MID-MORNING SNACK (106 MG SODIUM)

6 ounces fruit-flavored low-fat yogurt (105 mg sodium)

15 unsalted almonds (1 mg sodium)

LUNCH (392 MG SODIUM)

Green Soup with Goat Cheese* (270 mg sodium)

10 low-sodium whole-grain crackers (120 mg sodium)

1 cup diced pineapple (2 mg sodium)

MID-AFTERNOON SNACK (67 MG SODIUM)

2 stalks celery (64 mg sodium) with
- 1 tablespoon no-salt-added all-natural peanut butter (3 mg sodium)

DINNER (470 MG SODIUM)

Savory Turkey Meatloaf with Mushrooms* (390 mg sodium)

1 cup mashed sweet potatoes (40 mg sodium)

1 cup steamed broccoli and cauliflower (40 mg sodium)

DESSERT (79 MG SODIUM)

Lemon Meringue Layer Cake* (79 mg sodium)

Day 10 (1,376 mg sodium)

BREAKFAST (292 MG SODIUM)

Spicy Baked Eggs with Goat Cheese and Spinach* (260 mg sodium)
1 cup diced melon (30 mg sodium)
1 cup fresh orange juice (2 mg sodium)

MID-MORNING SNACK (177 MG SODIUM)

½ cup dried apricots (6 mg sodium)
1 (1-ounce) slice low-fat cheddar cheese (171 mg sodium)

LUNCH (445 MG SODIUM)

Caesar Salad Revamp* (343 mg sodium)
4 ounces cooked chicken breast (100 mg sodium)
1 medium pear (2 mg sodium)

MID-AFTERNOON SNACK (245 MG SODIUM)

3 gingersnaps (138 mg sodium)
1 cup 1 percent low-fat milk (107 mg sodium)

DINNER (131 MG SODIUM)

Balsamic-roasted chicken breast
- 1 (4-ounce) boneless, skinless chicken breast coated with 1 teaspoon olive oil and sprinkled with minced fresh rosemary, minced garlic, and freshly ground pepper, roasted at 450°F for about 20 minutes, turned once, and then drizzled with 1 tablespoon balsamic vinegar (131 mg sodium)

1 medium baked sweet potato (41 mg sodium)
Steamed green beans with squeeze of fresh lemon juice, 1 tablespoon unsalted butter, and 2 tablespoons slivered unsalted almonds

DESSERT (86 MG SODIUM)

1 medium apple, cored, filled with a mixture of 1 tablespoon unsalted butter, 1 tablespoon brown sugar, and ¼ teaspoon ground cinnamon, and baked in the microwave until soft (86 mg sodium)

Day 11 (1,385 mg sodium)

BREAKFAST (217 MG SODIUM)

1 whole-wheat English muffin with
- 1 tablespoon unsalted butter
- 1 tablespoon strawberry preserves (109 mg sodium)

1 cup fresh berries (1 mg sodium)
1 cup 1 percent low-fat milk (107 mg sodium)

MID-MORNING SNACK (11 MG SODIUM)

1 Chocolate Cherry Granola Bar* (11 mg sodium)

LUNCH (380 MG SODIUM)

Roasted Tomato Soup with Mint* (150 mg sodium)
1 slice toasted sourdough bread (220 mg sodium)
2 kiwifruits (10 mg sodium)

MID-AFTERNOON SNACK (34 MG SODIUM)

¼ cup unsalted dry-roasted pumpkin seeds (6 mg sodium)
1 cup diced cantaloupe (28 mg sodium)

DINNER (738 MG SODIUM)

Grilled Steak with Arugula and Lemon Vinaigrette* (674 mg sodium)
1 cup steamed broccoli (64 mg sodium)

DESSERT (5 MG SODIUM)

½ cup fruit sorbet (5 mg sodium)

Day 12 (1,491 mg sodium)

BREAKFAST (286 MG SODIUM)

Swiss Chard and Quinoa Frittata* (284 mg sodium)
1 cup diced fresh (or canned in juice) pineapple (2 mg sodium)

MID-MORNING SNACK (170 MG SODIUM)

½ cup part-skim ricotta cheese (170 mg sodium)
- ½ cup diced peaches or nectarines
- 2 teaspoons honey

LUNCH (472 MG SODIUM)

Hummus sandwich
- 1 whole-wheat pita (200 mg sodium)
- 2 tablespoons hummus (220 mg sodium)
- 1 tablespoon crumbled feta cheese (29 mg sodium)
- 1 cup shredded lettuce (10 mg sodium)
- 1 medium tomato, sliced (6 mg sodium)
1 cup snap peas (6 mg sodium)
1 medium orange (1 mg sodium)

MID-AFTERNOON SNACK (32 MG SODIUM)

1 unsalted brown rice cake (29 mg sodium) with
- 1 tablespoon no-salt-added all-natural peanut butter (3 mg sodium)

DINNER (527 MG SODIUM)

Spaghetti with Broiled Shrimp Scampi* (482 mg sodium)
1 cup sliced fennel bulb roasted with olive oil spray (45 mg sodium)

DESSERT (4 MG SODIUM)

1 cup sliced strawberries macerated in 2 teaspoons balsamic vinegar
(4 mg sodium)

Day 13 (1,496 mg sodium)

BREAKFAST (242 MG SODIUM)

Low-sodium instant oatmeal (72 mg sodium) with
- 1 tablespoon brown sugar (62 mg sodium)
- 1 cup blueberries (1 mg sodium)
- 1 cup 1 percent low-fat milk (107 mg sodium)

MID-MORNING SNACK (99 MG SODIUM)

1 apple-cinnamon rice cake (29 mg sodium) with
- 1 tablespoon light cream cheese (70 mg sodium)

LUNCH (438 MG SODIUM)

Roasted Beet Salad with Goat Cheese* (286 mg sodium)
1 medium pear (2 mg sodium)
½ whole-wheat roll (75 mg sodium)

MID-AFTERNOON SNACK (142 MG SODIUM)

6 ounces low-fat fruit-flavored yogurt (130 mg sodium)
1 tablespoon toasted rice cereal (12 mg sodium)

DINNER (573 MG SODIUM)

White Chicken Chili* (302 mg sodium)
- 1 ounce low-fat cheddar cheese, shredded (171 mg sodium)
- 1 green onion, thinly sliced (17 mg sodium)
1 tablespoon fresh salsa (75 mg sodium)
1 ounce unsalted baked tortilla chips (4 mg sodium)
½ cup grilled zucchini (4 mg sodium)

DESSERT (2 MG SODIUM)

1 cup mixed diced fruit: bananas, peaches, nectarines, pineapple, melon, berries (2 mg sodium)

Day 14 (1,115 mg sodium)

BREAKFAST (176 MG SODIUM)

1 whole-wheat English muffin (103 mg sodium)
1 egg, poached (70 mg sodium)
1 cup fresh orange juice (2 mg sodium)
1 medium banana (1 mg sodium)

MID-MORNING SNACK (3 MG SODIUM)

1 medium apple (2 mg sodium)
1 tablespoon no-salt-added almond butter (1 mg sodium)

LUNCH (454 MG SODIUM)

Greek salad with chickpeas
- 2 cups chopped romaine lettuce (8 mg sodium)
- ¼ cup canned chickpeas, drained and rinsed (156 mg sodium)
- 1 medium tomato, diced (6 mg sodium)
- ½ medium cucumber, diced (3 mg sodium)
- ¼ small red onion, thinly sliced (3 mg sodium)
- 2 tablespoons crumbled feta cheese (97 mg sodium)
- 1 tablespoon red wine vinegar mixed with 1 tablespoon olive oil (1 mg sodium)
1 ounce reduced-sodium pita chips (180 mg sodium)

MID-AFTERNOON SNACK (10 MG SODIUM)

1 ounce unsalted baked tortilla chips (4 mg sodium) with
- Fresh and Zingy Salsa Verde* (6 mg sodium)

DINNER (455 MG SODIUM)

Chinese-Style Beef and Vegetable Hot Pot* (445 mg sodium)
1 cup steamed brown rice, cooked without salt (10 mg sodium)

DESSERT (17 MG SODIUM)

1 Best Oatmeal-Chocolate Chip Cookie* (17 mg sodium)

PART TWO

Low-Sodium Recipes

CHAPTER SIX

Breakfasts

Everyone knows that breakfast is the most important meal of the day. It's too bad that so many breakfast foods—bacon, sausage, omelets, and more—are so often loaded with sodium. Not to worry, though. You can still enjoy your favorite breakfast foods even while you avoid excess sodium.

Here we've focused on breakfast recipes that are not only extremely nutritious but also filling, satisfying, and loaded with important nutrients instead of salt.

Rise and Shine Fruit Smoothie

SERVES 1

▶ *SODIUM //* **25 MG**

BUDGET-FRIENDLY // COOKING FOR ONE // LOW-FAT // QUICK

Fruit smoothies are the perfect grab-and-go breakfasts. They're delicious, packed with vitamins and antioxidants, and can be whipped up in just a couple of minutes. This one has creamy silken tofu for added protein to keep you going all morning. Drink it before you dash out the door, or take it along in a travel cup and drink it on the go.

1 cup frozen mixed berries
½ banana
½ cup fresh orange juice
¼ cup silken tofu

1. Combine all of the ingredients in a blender and process until smooth.

2. Pour the smoothie into a glass and serve immediately or transfer it to an insulated travel cup. Drink it within an hour.

Very Berry Breakfast Parfait

SERVES 4

▶ *SODIUM // **82 MG***

BUDGET-FRIENDLY // LOW-FAT // QUICK

Low in sodium, fat, and cholesterol and packed with vitamin C and calcium, these gorgeous parfaits are a perfect start to the day. They're so pretty and flavorful that you could even serve them as a healthful dessert.

1½ cups low-fat plain yogurt
3 tablespoons honey
1½ cups muesli breakfast cereal or low-sodium, low-fat granola
1½ cups mixed fresh berries (blackberries, raspberries, blueberries, or sliced
strawberries, in any combination)

1. Set out 4 parfait glasses, 8-ounce mason jars, or other 8-ounce glasses.

2. In a small mixing bowl, combine the yogurt and honey and stir to mix well.

3. Spoon 2 tablespoons of the yogurt mixture into the bottom of each glass or jar. Top with 2 tablespoons of the cereal, and then 2 tablespoons of the fruit. Repeat until all of the ingredients have been used.

4. Serve immediately or cover and refrigerate the parfaits for up to 2 hours.

Cherry-Almond Granola

SERVES 8

▶ *SODIUM //* **81 MG**

MAKE AHEAD

Homemade granola is always a crowd-pleaser, and it's so easy to make. This version is sweetened with a combination of apple juice and maple syrup and gets an extra boost of fiber from wheat germ and flaxseed. Cherries, almonds, and coconut give it plenty of flavor.

....

Cooking spray

⅓ cup frozen unsweetened apple juice from concentrate, thawed

¼ cup maple syrup

3 tablespoons canola oil

2 tablespoons brown sugar

1 teaspoon vanilla extract

2½ cups old-fashioned quick-cooking rolled oats

½ cup toasted wheat germ

½ cup sliced almonds

½ cup shredded unsweetened coconut

2 tablespoons ground flaxseed

½ cup chopped dried cherries

....

1. Preheat the oven to 325°F.

2. Position an oven rack in the middle of the oven and spray a large baking sheet with cooking spray.

3. In a medium saucepan set over medium-high heat, combine the apple juice, maple syrup, oil, and brown sugar and cook, stirring occasionally, for 3 to 5 minutes, or until the sugar is dissolved. Remove the saucepan from the heat and stir in the vanilla.

4. In a large bowl, combine the oats, wheat germ, almonds, coconut, and flaxseed. Pour in the liquid from the saucepan and stir to coat well. Spread the mixture on the prepared baking sheet.

5. Bake the granola in the oven for 15 minutes, and then remove the baking sheet from the oven and stir the granola.

6. Put the baking sheet back in the oven, rotating it from front to back. Bake for about 15 minutes more, stirring several times, until the granola begins to brown.

7. Remove the granola from the oven and stir in the cherries. Let it cool to room temperature on the baking sheet, and then transfer the granola to a glass jar to store.

8. Serve the granola at room temperature with nonfat or low-fat milk, or nonfat yogurt.

Creamy Strawberry Oatmeal

SERVES 1

▶ *SODIUM //* **77 MG**

BUDGET-FRIENDLY // COOKING FOR ONE // LOW-FAT // QUICK

Oatmeal is full of fiber, which keeps you feeling full but also reduces cholesterol and limits your risk for numerous diseases, including diabetes, high blood pressure, heart disease, and cancer. This version is creamy, sweet, and loaded with vitamin C. Feel free to substitute other fruits, such as peaches, bananas, or pears, as the seasons change.

....

½ cup water

¼ cup low-fat milk

½ cup old-fashioned quick-cooking rolled oats

½ cup sliced strawberries

¼ cup nonfat Greek yogurt

1 tablespoon honey

....

1. In a small saucepan set over medium heat, combine the water, milk, and oats. Bring the mixture to a boil, stirring occasionally.

2. Once the mixture is boiling, reduce the heat to low and simmer for 3 to 5 minutes, stirring occasionally, until the oats are tender.

3. Remove from the heat, cover, and let stand for 3 to 5 minutes.

4. Spoon the oatmeal into a serving bowl. Stir in the strawberries, yogurt, and honey and serve immediately.

Lemon-Blueberry Muffins

MAKES 12 MUFFINS

▶ *SODIUM* // **133 MG** *(PER MUFFIN)*
BUDGET-FRIENDLY // LOW-FAT // MAKE AHEAD

Low-fat buttermilk makes these muffins super-moist and gives them a rich, tangy flavor. Make these muffins when antioxidant-rich blueberries are at their peak of ripeness in the summer, or any time of year using frozen berries (they'll be just as delicious!).

Cooking spray (optional)
1 cup whole-wheat flour
1 cup all-purpose flour
2 teaspoons baking powder
1 teaspoon baking soda
½ cup sugar
Zest of 1 lemon
1 cup low-fat buttermilk
⅓ cup canola oil
1 egg
1 teaspoon vanilla extract
1½ cups fresh or frozen (not thawed) blueberries

1. Preheat the oven to 400°F.

2. Line a standard 12-cup muffin tin with paper liners or spray it with nonstick cooking spray.

3. In a medium mixing bowl, combine the flours, baking powder, and baking soda.

4. Place the sugar in large mixing bowl. Using the fine holes of a cheese grater or a Microplane grater, zest the lemon directly into the bowl with the sugar. Stir to combine.

continued ▶

5. Add the buttermilk, oil, egg, and vanilla and beat using an electric mixer on medium speed until well combined.

6. Add the dry ingredients to the wet ingredients in 2 or 3 batches, beating just to combine after each addition.

7. Gently fold in the blueberries.

8. Spoon the batter into the prepared muffin tin, dividing it equally. Bake in the oven for 20 to 25 minutes, until the tops are golden and a toothpick inserted into the center comes out clean.

9. Let the muffins cool in the pan for a few minutes before transferring them to a wire rack. Serve warm or at room temperature.

Healthful Apple Muffins with Cinnamon-Pecan Topping

MAKES 12 MUFFINS

▶ *SODIUM //* **136 MG** *(PER MUFFIN)*
BUDGET-FRIENDLY // MAKE AHEAD

Apples and cinnamon go together like peanut butter and jelly. Applesauce makes these muffins moist without a lot of added fat, and the crunchy pecan topping turns them into a real treat.

For the topping:
¼ cup chopped pecans
2 tablespoons brown sugar
½ teaspoon ground cinnamon

For the muffins:
Cooking spray (optional)
1 cup all-purpose flour
1 cup whole-wheat pastry flour
1 teaspoon baking soda
¼ teaspoon ground cinnamon
¾ cup packed brown sugar
¼ cup canola oil
2 eggs
1 cup unsweetened applesauce
1 teaspoon vanilla extract
¾ cup low-fat buttermilk
1 medium apple, peeled, cored, and cut into ¼-inch dice

To make the topping:

1. In a small bowl, mix together the pecans, brown sugar, and cinnamon.

continued ▶

To make the muffins:

1. Preheat the oven to 400°F.

2. Line a standard 12-cup muffin tin with paper liners or spray it with nonstick cooking spray.

3. In a medium mixing bowl, combine the flours, baking soda, and cinnamon.

4. In a large bowl, combine the brown sugar and oil.

5. Add the eggs, one at a time, whisking after each addition until the eggs are incorporated.

6. Stir in the applesauce and vanilla.

7. Add half of the flour mixture and stir to combine. Add half of the buttermilk and the remaining flour, stirring again until combined. Add the remaining buttermilk and stir to combine.

8. Fold in the apple.

9. Spoon the batter into the prepared muffin tin, dividing equally. Sprinkle the nut topping over the top. Bake in the oven for 20 to 25 minutes, until a toothpick inserted into the center comes out clean.

10. Place the pan on a wire rack and allow it to cool for about 10 minutes. Transfer the muffins to the wire rack and allow them cool completely. Serve at room temperature.

Maple-Cinnamon Oatmeal Pancakes

SERVES 4

▸ *SODIUM //* **130 MG**

BUDGET-FRIENDLY // LOW-FAT // QUICK

Low-fat buttermilk adds a ton of flavor and protein to these healthful, fiber-filled pancakes. Serve them with fresh fruit, yogurt, powdered sugar, or drizzled with additional maple syrup.

1½ cups old-fashioned quick-cooking rolled oats
½ cup whole-wheat flour
1 teaspoon ground cinnamon
1 teaspoon baking powder
2 cups low-fat buttermilk
2 tablespoons maple syrup
1 egg
Cooking spray

1. In a medium mixing bowl, combine the oats, flour, cinnamon, and baking powder.

2. In a large mixing bowl, whisk together the buttermilk, maple syrup, and egg.

3. Add the dry mixture to the wet mixture in 2 or 3 additions, mixing well after each addition. Let it stand for 10 to 15 minutes, until the mixture becomes bubbly.

4. Spray a nonstick skillet with cooking spray and heat it over medium heat. Spoon the batter into the pan, about ¼ cup for each pancake, and cook for 2 to 3 minutes, until bubbles appear on the surface. Flip and continue to cook another 1 to 2 minutes, until each pancake is browned on the second side.

5. Cook in batches of 3 or 4 (depending on the size of your pan) until you use up all of the batter. Serve immediately.

Swiss Chard and Quinoa Frittata

SERVES 6

▸ *SODIUM //* **284 MG**

BUDGET-FRIENDLY

Packed with protein, this is a real power breakfast. The greens add plenty of vitamins A and C, and each serving delivers nearly six grams of fiber, too, which will keep you feeling full until lunchtime.

....

Cooking spray
⅓ cup unseasoned bread crumbs
1 tablespoon olive oil
1 medium onion, diced
2 garlic cloves, minced
1 pound Swiss chard leaves, tough center stem removed and leaves thinly sliced
1 tablespoon minced fresh thyme, or 1 teaspoon dried thyme
¼ teaspoon red pepper flakes
1 cup quinoa, cooked according to package directions (about 2 cups cooked)
1 cup part-skim ricotta cheese
¼ teaspoon freshly ground pepper
2 eggs, lightly beaten

....

1. Preheat the oven to 350°F.

2. Spray an an 8 by 8-inch baking dish with cooking spray and coat it with the bread crumbs.

3. Heat the oil in a large skillet over medium-high heat. Add the onion and garlic and cook, stirring frequently, until softened, about 5 minutes.

4. Add the chard and cook another 3 to 4 minutes, stirring frequently, until the greens are wilted. Stir in the thyme and red pepper flakes.

5. Remove the skillet from the heat and transfer the chard mixture to a medium mixing bowl.

6. Stir the cooked quinoa, cheese, pepper, and eggs into the chard mixture. Transfer the mixture to the prepared baking dish, and bake in the oven for about 1 hour, until the edges are just beginning to brown and the center is set.

7. Let the frittata cool for a few minutes before cutting it into squares. Serve warm or at room temperature.

Spicy Baked Eggs with Goat Cheese and Spinach

SERVES 4

▸ *SODIUM //* **260 MG**
QUICK

Loaded with iron from the spinach, these eggs can be made even spicier with a hot salsa. These are quick and easy, and make a great breakfast on a busy morning.

Cooking spray
10 ounces frozen chopped spinach, thawed and squeezed dry
4 eggs
¼ cup chunky salsa
¼ cup crumbled goat cheese
Freshly ground pepper

1. Preheat the oven to 325°F.

2. Spray four 6-ounce ramekins or custard cups with cooking spray.

3. Cover the bottom of each ramekin with spinach, dividing it equally. Make a slight indentation in the center of each layer of spinach.

4. Crack one egg on top of the spinach in each ramekin. Top each egg with 1 tablespoon of salsa and 1 tablespoon of goat cheese. Sprinkle with pepper.

5. Place the ramekins on a baking sheet and bake in the oven for about 20 minutes, until the whites are completely set, but the yolk is still a bit runny. Serve immediately.

Garlicky Mushroom and Cheese Omelet

SERVES 1

▸ *SODIUM //* **200 MG**

BUDGET-FRIENDLY // COOKING FOR ONE // QUICK

Omelets are quick and easy to make and there are endless variations. This one is full of garlicky sautéed mushrooms and Swiss cheese. Using low-fat, low-sodium cheese keeps it healthful. It's a hearty breakfast that's fast enough to make on a weekday morning but special enough to serve for brunch.

2 eggs

1 teaspoon water

Freshly ground pepper

Cooking spray

½ teaspoon minced garlic

4 ounces sliced button or cremini mushrooms

1 ounce shredded low-fat, low-sodium Swiss cheese

1 teaspoon minced fresh parsley

1. In a small bowl, whisk the eggs, water, and pepper to taste together until well combined.

2. Spray a small nonstick skillet with cooking spray and heat it over medium heat. Add the garlic and mushrooms and cook, stirring frequently, until the mushrooms are soft, about 5 minutes. Transfer the mushroom mixture to a bowl.

3. Spray the skillet again with cooking spray, if needed, and place it over medium heat. Add the eggs and cook them until the edges begin to set. With a spatula, push the set egg from the edges toward the center. Tilt the pan, allowing the uncooked egg to spread around the outside of the set egg. Cook until the omelet is nearly set.

continued ▸

4. Spoon the cooked mushrooms into the omelet in a line down the center. Top with the cheese and half of the parsley.

5. Fold one side of the omelet over the top of the other side. Let it cook for 1 minute or so more to melt the cheese.

6. Slide the omelet onto a plate and serve immediately, garnished with the remaining parsley.

CHAPTER SEVEN

Snacks and Appetizers

S o often, the snacks and appetizers we reach for are full of fat, sugar, and sodium because when we are feeling peckish in the middle of the workday, craving nibbles while watching a game on TV, or hungry just before mealtime, what we really want is tons of flavor. And let's face it: fat, sugar, and salt deliver lots of flavor in satisfying morsels.

In this chapter, we've provided recipes for quick snacks, sweet treats, and crave-worthy appetizers that skimp on fat, sugar, and salt but not on flavor. So go ahead and snack without guilt or regrets.

Lemon-Pepper Popcorn with Parmesan

SERVES 4

▸ *SODIUM //* **105 MG**
LOW-FAT // QUICK

You might not think of popcorn as a health food, but it is a whole grain. It is full of fiber and loaded with disease-fighting antioxidants. The big problem is that people tend to cook it in oil, drench it with butter, and load it with salt. In this version, we start with low-fat air-popped popcorn and add lots of flavor with lemon pepper and a bit of grated Parmesan cheese. So go ahead, mix up a batch for your next movie night.

4 cups air-popped popcorn
2 tablespoons grated Parmesan cheese
¾ teaspoon lemon pepper seasoning

1. In a large bowl, combine all of the ingredients. Toss well and serve immediately.

Curry-Lime Peanuts

SERVES 8

▶ *SODIUM //* **155 MG**

BUDGET-FRIENDLY // MAKE AHEAD

Peanuts are a great source of heart-healthful monounsaturated fats as well as vitamins and minerals—including vitamin E, niacin, folate, and manganese— that are known to promote a healthy heart. They also deliver high doses of resveratrol, the antioxidant that gives red wine its reputation as a heart-healthful beverage.

2 tablespoons fresh lime juice

2 tablespoons curry powder

¼ teaspoon cayenne pepper (optional)

2 cups unsalted peanuts

1. Preheat the oven to 250°F.

2. In a medium mixing bowl, whisk together the lime juice, curry powder, and cayenne, if using, until well combined. Add the peanuts and stir to coat.

3. Spread the peanuts in an even layer on a large baking sheet.

4. Bake the peanuts in the oven, stirring occasionally, for 45 to 50 minutes, until they begin to brown.

5. Allow the peanuts to cool completely before eating; they can be stored in an airtight container at room temperature for up to 1 week.

Oven-Baked Rosemary Sweet Potato Chips

SERVES 2

▸ *SODIUM //* **33 MG**

BUDGET-FRIENDLY // COOKING FOR TWO // LOW-FAT // QUICK

Regular potato chips are packed with sodium and offer little in the way of nutrition, but we all know just how crave-worthy they are. The next time you are gripped with an uncontrollable chip craving, try this much healthier version. Sweet potatoes are loaded with vitamins B_6, C, and D as well as minerals like potassium and magnesium, which is essential for healthful heart function. Their bright orange color is proof that they are full of beta-carotenes, which reduce the risk of many diseases, including cancer, and fight the effects of aging. A mandoline is the best tool for getting really thin and uniform slices, but a food processor or just a sharp knife and a bit of patience will work, too.

Cooking spray
1 large sweet potato, peeled and thinly sliced
1 teaspoon minced fresh rosemary

1. Preheat the oven to 400°F.

2. Coat 2 large baking sheets with cooking spray.

3. Arrange the potato slices on the prepared baking sheets in a single layer. Spray them with cooking spray and sprinkle them with the rosemary.

4. Bake one sheet at a time in the oven for about 15 minutes, until the chips just begin to brown. Transfer the chips to a rack to cool.

5. Serve immediately or store the chips in an airtight container at room temperature for up to 2 days.

Jalapeño-Cilantro Hummus

SERVES 6

▶ *SODIUM //* **24 MG**

BUDGET-FRIENDLY // LOW-FAT // QUICK

Store-bought hummus, while full of protein, fiber, vitamins, and minerals, is usually sodium-heavy. This homemade version is quick to make and relies on fresh chilies and cilantro, instead of salt, for flavor. Serve this tasty dip with crudités or whole-wheat pita triangles for a healthful snack or appetizer.

1 (15-ounce) can chickpeas, drained and rinsed
1 cup cilantro leaves, plus additional for garnish
2 small jalapeños, seeded and coarsely chopped
1 garlic clove
¼ cup fresh lime juice
2 tablespoons tahini (sesame paste)
1 tablespoon olive oil

1. In a food processor, puree the chickpeas, cilantro, jalapeños, and garlic until smooth.

2. Add the lime juice, tahini, and oil and process until well blended. If the mixture is too thick, add water, 1 tablespoon at a time, until the desired consistency is achieved.

3. Serve the hummus immediately, garnished with additional cilantro, or cover and refrigerate it for up to 2 days.

Fresh Garlic and Herb Yogurt Dip

SERVES 8

▶ *SODIUM //* **50 MG**
LOW-FAT // QUICK

Who doesn't love a creamy onion dip with crispy potato chips? This yogurt-based version is loaded with herbs and fresh garlic, keeping it healthful, light, and delicious. Serve it with our Oven-Baked Rosemary Sweet Potato Chips (page 36) or fresh vegetable crudités for a satisfying snack.

1 cup nonfat Greek yogurt
½ cup grated cucumber, drained and squeezed dry
2 tablespoons grated yellow onion
1 tablespoon fresh lemon juice
1 tablespoon minced fresh dill
1 tablespoon minced fresh mint
1 teaspoon minced fresh oregano
2 teaspoons honey
2 garlic cloves, minced
1 teaspoon olive oil

1. In a medium bowl, combine all of the ingredients. Stir to mix well.

2. Cover and refrigerate the dip for at least 1 hour to allow the flavors to meld.

3. Serve the dip immediately or store it in the refrigerator for up to 2 days.

Sweet Pea and Ricotta Toasts

SERVES 8

▸ *SODIUM //* **467 MG**

BUDGET-FRIENDLY // LOW-FAT // QUICK

The bright green of the pea puree indicates its super-healthful qualities. In addition to protein and fiber, peas are full of antioxidants. Here they are paired with creamy ricotta cheese, lemon, and basil for a pretty appetizer that would be perfect for a spring dinner party but can be made, with frozen peas, any time of year.

....

1½ cups frozen peas
Juice of 1 lemon
1 tablespoon olive oil
½ cup chopped fresh basil, plus additional for garnish
½ teaspoon freshly ground pepper, plus additional for garnish
24 thin slices whole-wheat baguette
Cooking spray
1 garlic clove, halved
¾ cup part-skim ricotta cheese

....

1. Preheat the oven to 400°F.

2. Cook the peas until tender according to the package instructions. Drain and rinse the peas with cold water.

3. Place the cooked peas, lemon juice, oil, basil, and pepper in a food processor and process until smooth.

4. Spray the baguette slices with cooking spray and arrange them in a single layer on a large baking sheet. Bake the baguette slices in the oven for 4 to 5 minutes per side, until the bread is crisp and golden brown.

5. Remove the baguette slices from the oven and let them cool for several minutes on a wire rack.

continued ▶

6. Rub each piece of toast with the cut sides of the halved garlic clove.

7. Preheat the broiler.

8. Spread the ricotta cheese on the toasted baguette slices and arrange them on the baking sheet. Broil for 1 to 2 minutes, until the cheese is warm and begins to bubble.

9. Top each toast with a dollop of the pea puree, garnish with freshly ground pepper and minced basil, and serve immediately.

Zesty Sun-Dried Tomato and Bacon Bread Twists

MAKES 8 TWISTS

▸ *SODIUM //* **150 MG** *(PER TWIST)*
LOW-FAT // QUICK

Bacon is one of those foods that many people find especially hard to give up when health concerns force them to restrict their diet. So rich and delicious, bacon is fantastic on its own and adds depth of flavor to so many dishes. Here we've substituted healthier turkey bacon and used just a couple of slices. The crumbled bits are sprinkled throughout these tantalizing bread sticks, distributing the flavor through every twist.

....

2 tablespoons chopped sun-dried tomatoes

½ cup all-purpose flour

¼ cup whole-wheat flour

1 teaspoon low-sodium baking powder

¼ teaspoon red pepper flakes

⅛ teaspoon cream of tartar

2½ tablespoons unsalted butter

2 slices turkey bacon, cooked and crumbled

¼ cup nonfat milk

Cooking spray

2 tablespoons grated Parmesan cheese

....

1. Preheat the oven to 425°F.

2. In a small bowl, cover the sun-dried tomatoes with hot water and let them sit for 5 minutes to reconstitute the tomatoes. Drain, discarding the soaking liquid.

continued ▸

3. In a food processor, combine the flours, baking powder, red pepper flakes, and cream of tartar. Add the butter and pulse until the mixture resembles a coarse meal. Transfer the mixture to a medium mixing bowl.

4. Stir in the bacon and tomatoes. Add the milk and stir just until the dough comes together.

5. Turn the dough out onto a lightly floured work surface and knead it several times, until it becomes smooth. Pat the dough out into a 4 by 4-inch square.

6. Cut the square into 4 equal strips and then halve each strip crosswise. Twist each strip and lay it on a large baking sheet.

7. Spray the bread twists with cooking spray, sprinkle with the cheese, and bake in the oven until a light golden brown, about 10 minutes. Serve immediately.

Crabmeat Quesadillas

SERVES 6

▶ *SODIUM //* **450 MG**
QUICK

Low-calorie crab provides lots of protein and nutrients, including vitamins B$_{12}$ and C, as well as omega-3 fatty acids, which help to prevent heart disease. These spicy wedges are the perfect snack to serve while watching a football game or as an appetizer before a Mexican-style dinner.

¾ cup shredded low-sodium cheddar cheese
2 ounces reduced-fat cream cheese, softened
4 green onions, thinly sliced
½ medium red bell pepper, finely chopped
⅓ cup chopped cilantro
1 jalapeño, seeded and minced
1 teaspoon lime zest
1 tablespoon fresh lime juice
8 ounces lump crabmeat
4 whole-wheat flour tortillas
Cooking spray

1. In a medium bowl, stir together the cheddar cheese, cream cheese, green onions, bell pepper, cilantro, jalapeño, lime zest, and lime juice. Fold in the crabmeat, being careful not to break it up too much.

2. Spread the crabmeat mixture onto one half of each of the tortillas, dividing it evenly. Fold the tortillas over to make half-moons.

3. Spray a large nonstick skillet with cooking spray and heat it over medium heat. Cook 2 quesadillas at a time, for about 3 minutes per side, until they are golden brown and the filling is hot.

4. Remove the quesadillas from the pan and keep them warm while you cook the remaining quesadillas.

5. Cut each quesadilla into 4 wedges and serve warm.

Frozen Yogurt-Berry Buttons

SERVES 1

▸ *SODIUM //* **103 MG**

BUDGET-FRIENDLY // COOKING FOR ONE // LOW-FAT

Sometimes you just need a little sweet treat in the middle of the day. These tasty little yogurt drops are the perfect thing. They are made with nonfat yogurt, berries, and just a touch of honey, so they are perfectly healthful, but they satisfy that midday sugar craving like nobody's business. The recipe can be easily doubled, tripled, or quadrupled, and the drops can be stored in the freezer for up to three months, but it's unlikely they'll be around anywhere near that long.

½ cup frozen mixed berries
1 cup nonfat plain Greek yogurt
1 teaspoon honey

1. Line a baking sheet with parchment paper (make sure the baking sheet will fit in your freezer).

2. In a food processor or blender, puree the berries. Add the yogurt and honey and process until smooth and well combined.

3. Drop the yogurt-berry mixture by ¼ teaspoonfuls onto the parchment paper, leaving space in between so that they don't spread into one another.

4. Place the baking sheet in the freezer and freeze until the drops are solid, at least 3 hours.

5. Serve immediately, or transfer the drops to a freezer-safe, sealable plastic bag and store until ready to eat.

Chocolate Cherry Granola Bars

MAKES 12 BARS

▸ *SODIUM //* **11 MG** *(PER BAR)*
LOW-FAT // MAKE AHEAD

Dark chocolate and dried cherries are both super foods that are loaded with disease-fighting antioxidants. Flaxseed, too, adds extra fiber and nutrients as well as a nice nutty crunch.

Cooking spray
2 cups old-fashioned quick-cooking rolled oats
1 cup slivered almonds
¼ cup flaxseed
⅔ cup honey
¼ cup packed brown sugar
3 tablespoons coconut oil
1½ teaspoons vanilla extract
½ cup chopped dried cherries
½ cup chopped dark chocolate

1. Preheat the oven to 350°F.

2. Spray an an 8 by 12-inch baking pan with cooking spray.

3. In a large mixing bowl, combine the oats and almonds and stir to mix well. Spread the mixture out on a large baking sheet and bake in the oven for about 10 minutes, stirring occasionally, until lightly toasted.

4. Return the mixture to the large mixing bowl and stir in the flaxseed.

5. Reduce the oven temperature to 300°F.

6. In a small saucepan set over medium heat, combine the honey, brown sugar, and coconut oil and bring to a boil. Cook, stirring, for 1 minute, and then stir in the vanilla.

continued ▸

7. Add the honey mixture to the oat mixture mixture along with the cherries and stir well. Fold in the chocolate.

8. Transfer the mixture into the prepared baking pan. Press the mixture into an even layer in the pan. Bake the granola in the oven for 25 to 28 minutes, until the granola begins to brown.

9. Remove the pan from the oven and set it on a rack to cool to room temperature.

10. Cut the granola into 12 bars and serve at room temperature, or store them in an airtight container at room temperature for up to 1 week.

CHAPTER EIGHT

Condiments and Sauces

C ondiments and sauces are often the downfall of even the best intentioned among us. These tasty sauces, spreads, dips, and dressings are often full of hidden sodium, not to mention saturated fat, sugar, and other undesirable ingredients. By making your own condiments at home, you can be sure that they contain only good-for-you ingredients—or at least only limited amounts of the naughty ones.

From ketchup to mayonnaise, barbecue sauce, pasta sauce, and even spicy Asian dipping sauces, this chapter provides simple recipes for do-it-yourself versions of the most popular condiments and sauces. Get out your spoon, knife, or baked French fry and get to spreading, saucing, and dipping to your heart's content.

Double-Tomato Ketchup

MAKES 2 CUPS (1 TABLESPOON PER SERVING)

▸ *SODIUM //* **46 MG** *(PER TABLESPOON)*
LOW-FAT // MAKE AHEAD // QUICK

This homemade version of that ubiquitous American condiment gets a double dose of rich tomato flavor from both tomato paste and sun-dried tomatoes. You may not be able to claim a serving of ketchup as one of your five veggie servings for the day with a clean conscience, but you can rest assured that you'll get a hefty boost of vitamins B_6 and C as well as thiamine, niacin, phosphorous, and copper. Plus, homemade ketchup adds irresistible flavor to all kinds of healthful foods, like baked French fries or sweet potato fries, turkey burgers, and hash browns.

2 (6-ounce) cans tomato paste
⅔ cup water
¼ cup red wine vinegar
½ cup packed dark brown sugar
¼ cup chopped sun-dried tomatoes
½ teaspoon dry mustard
½ teaspoon cinnamon
⅛ teaspoon ground cloves
⅛ teaspoon allspice
Pinch of cayenne pepper

1. In a saucepan set over medium heat, whisk together all of the ingredients and bring to a simmer. Cook, stirring, until the sugar has dissolved. Reduce the heat to low and simmer for about 15 minutes.

2. Remove the mixture from the heat and puree it in a blender or food processor.

3. Allow it to cool to room temperature. Cover and refrigerate the ketchup overnight before serving. Ketchup can be refrigerated for up to 3 weeks.

Sweet-Spicy Red Pepper Relish

SERVES 20 (MAKES 2½ CUPS, 2 TABLESPOONS PER SERVING)

▸ *SODIUM //* **59 MG** *(PER 2 TABLESPOONS)*
LOW-FAT // MAKE AHEAD

This sweet, tangy, and peppery relish is a perfect match for hotdogs, hamburgers, and anything else you'd normally put a sweet pickle relish on. A food processor makes quick work of shredding the onions and bell peppers, but a box grater will work as well.

2 large yellow onions, finely shredded
2 medium red bell peppers, seeded and finely shredded
1 cup sugar
½ cup white wine vinegar
¼ cup water
½ teaspoon red pepper flakes

1. In a large saucepan set over medium-high heat, combine all of the ingredients and bring to a boil. Reduce the heat to low and simmer, uncovered, for about 30 minutes, stirring often, until the vegetables are very soft and the mixture is well combined.

2. Remove the relish from the heat and allow it to cool to room temperature.

3. Cover and refrigerate the relish for at least 2 hours before serving. Store it in a covered container in the refrigerator for up to 1 month.

Barbecue Sauce

SERVES 16 (MAKES 2 CUPS, 2 TABLESPOONS PER SERVING)

▸ *SODIUM //* **34 MG** *(PER 2 TABLESPOONS)*
LOW-FAT // MAKE AHEAD // QUICK

Barbecue sauce is one of the sneakiest condiments when it comes to salt, but this version is so full of flavor, we're certain you won't miss the salt we've eliminated.

1½ cups no-salt-added tomato sauce
1 (6-ounce) can tomato paste
⅔ cup packed dark brown sugar
3 tablespoons apple cider vinegar
1½ tablespoons molasses
1 tablespoon Worcestershire sauce
1 tablespoon smoked paprika
2 teaspoons dry mustard
2 teaspoons chili powder
1 teaspoon onion powder
½ teaspoon liquid smoke (optional)
½ teaspoon garlic powder
¼ teaspoon ground cloves
¼ teaspoon cayenne pepper

1. Combine all of the ingredients in a medium saucepan over medium-high heat. Bring to a boil, reduce the heat to medium-low, and simmer, stirring occasionally, for 20 to 30 minutes, until the sauce is slightly thickened.

2. Serve the sauce immediately or allow it to cool to room temperature, transfer it to a covered container, and refrigerate it for up to 1 month.

Creamy Lemon-Chive Sandwich Spread

SERVES 16 (MAKES 1 CUP, 1 TABLESPOON PER SERVING)

▶ *SODIUM //* **16 MG** *(PER TABLESPOON)*
LOW-FAT // MAKE AHEAD // QUICK

This tangy-creamy sauce is a great stand-in for mayonnaise on sandwiches. Made with a combination of nonfat sour cream and reduced-fat mayo, it has all the rich spreadability you want in a sandwich spread, but with very little fat and sodium. Lemon juice and zest add a burst of bright citrus flavor, and chopped chives provide a fresh, herby element. Add a few spoonfuls of minced low-sodium pickles and it becomes a wonderful tartar sauce, too.

½ cup nonfat sour cream
¼ cup reduced-fat mayonnaise
3 tablespoons chopped chives
1½ teaspoons lemon zest
2 teaspoons fresh lemon juice

1. In a small bowl, whisk all of the ingredients together until well combined. Serve immediately or cover and refrigerate the spread for up to 3 days.

Basil-Cilantro Pesto

SERVES 8 (MAKES ABOUT 1 CUP, 2 TABLESPOONS PER SERVING)

▶ *SODIUM //* **37 MG** *(PER 2 TABLESPOONS)*
LOW-FAT // MAKE AHEAD // QUICK

Both basil and cilantro are considered cleansing herbs, offering antibacterial and antifungal properties. They are rich in vitamins, minerals, and antioxidants that are essential for healthful organ function, too. Better still, they taste fantastic. Serve this pesto as a sauce for pasta, a spread for bread on sandwiches, or on roasted or grilled chicken, fish, or vegetables. If you don't care for cilantro, substitute mint or arugula.

2 tablespoons pine nuts
1 cup fresh basil leaves
1 cup fresh cilantro leaves
1 garlic clove
¼ cup low-sodium chicken broth
2 tablespoons olive oil
2 tablespoons fresh lemon juice
¼ cup grated Parmesan cheese

1. Toast the pine nuts in a skillet over medium heat, stirring frequently, just until they begin to turn golden and become aromatic, about 3 minutes.

2. In a food processor, combine the pine nuts, basil, cilantro, and garlic. Process until smooth.

3. Add the broth, oil, and lemon juice and process to a thick paste. Add the cheese and pulse to combine.

4. Serve immediately or cover and refrigerate the pesto for up to 3 days. Pesto keeps best if a thin film of oil is poured over the surface to keep the herbs from oxidizing too quickly.

Fresh Tomato-Basil Pasta Sauce

SERVES 4 (MAKES 2 CUPS, ½ CUP PER SERVING)

▸ *SODIUM //* **43 MG** *(PER ½ CUP)*
BUDGET-FRIENDLY // LOW-FAT // QUICK

Few things are more satisfying than a bowl of pasta with a bright, fresh tomato sauce flecked with garlic and basil. If you take a few minutes to make this sauce, you'll be glad you did. Make this sauce in the summertime when both tomatoes and basil are at their peak.

2¼ pounds plum tomatoes
2 tablespoons olive oil
6 to 8 garlic cloves, minced
2 medium onions, diced
2 tablespoons tomato paste
¼ cup red wine
1 tablespoon red wine vinegar
½ cup chopped fresh basil
Freshly ground pepper

1. Place a large stockpot full of water on the stove and bring it to a boil over high heat. Fill a large mixing bowl with ice water.

2. Meanwhile, score an X in the bottom of each tomato with a sharp knife. Blanch the tomatoes in the boiling water for about 1 minute—you may have to do this in batches, using a slotted spoon to remove the blanched tomatoes.

3. Transfer the tomatoes from the boiling water to the bowl of ice water to stop the cooking.

4. When cool, peel off the skins with a paring knife (they should slip off easily). Halve and seed the tomatoes and coarsely chop the flesh, retaining any juice.

continued ▶

5. Heat the oil in a large, heavy pot set over medium heat. Add the garlic and onion and cook, stirring occasionally, until the onions are soft, about 5 minutes.

6. Stir in the tomato paste and cook for about 2 minutes.

7. Add the wine and vinegar and cook, stirring, for another 2 minutes.

8. Add the tomatoes and their juice and simmer, stirring occasionally, for about 20 minutes.

9. Stir in the basil, season with pepper, and puree using an immersion blender or by transferring to a blender in batches.

10. Serve immediately over cooked pasta or refrigerate the sauce in a covered container for up to 1 week.

Bolognese Sauce

SERVES 4

▸ *SODIUM //* **220 MG**

BUDGET-FRIENDLY // MAKE AHEAD

We've cut the salt but left all the tomato-rich, meaty flavor. This sauce is perfect on pasta or a bowl of smooth, hearty polenta. Make a double (or triple!) batch and freeze some for another day.

2 tablespoons olive oil

2 small yellow onions, finely chopped

2 medium carrots, diced small

2 stalks celery, diced small

1½ pounds lean ground beef

1½ cups red wine

1 cup low-fat milk

3 (14-ounce) cans no-salt-added diced tomatoes, with juice

¼ teaspoon ground nutmeg

1. In a large, heavy pot, heat the oil over medium-high heat. Add the onions, carrots, and celery and cook, stirring occasionally, for about 10 minutes, until the vegetables are tender.

2. Add the meat and cook, stirring and breaking up the meat with a wooden spoon, until the meat is completely browned, about 5 minutes.

3. Stir in the wine and cook, stirring occasionally, for 20 to 25 minutes, until most of the liquid has evaporated.

4. Stir in the milk and continue to cook, stirring occasionally, for another 15 minutes, until the milk has been mostly reduced.

5. Add the tomatoes, along with their juice, and the nutmeg, and bring to a boil. Reduce the heat to medium-low and simmer, uncovered, for 3 to 4 hours. The sauce is ready when it is thick and most of the liquid has evaporated.

6. Serve immediately or store the sauce in a covered container in the refrigerator for up to 3 days, or in the freezer for up to 3 months.

Spicy Peanut Sauce

SERVES 8

▸ *SODIUM //* **141 MG**
MAKE AHEAD // QUICK

Peanuts are high in protein and healthful fats, but that's not all. They also deliver a wallop of resveratrol, the same antioxidant that gives red wine its famous heart-protecting and cancer-preventing qualities. They are also high in phytosterols, which help to promote healthful cholesterol levels and protect against heart disease. Once you taste this spicy-sweet-savory sauce, you'll want to put it on everything. It's a natural topping for noodles, grilled meats, and roasted vegetables. You can even add a bit of extra lemon juice or rice vinegar to turn it into a fantastic salad dressing.

1 (1-inch) piece fresh ginger, peeled and coarsely chopped
1 garlic clove, minced
⅔ cup unsalted creamy peanut butter
3 tablespoons low-sodium soy sauce
3 tablespoons unseasoned rice vinegar
2 tablespoons packed brown sugar
2 teaspoons toasted sesame oil
¼ teaspoon cayenne pepper, or more, if desired
2 to 3 tablespoons water, as needed

1. Place the ginger and garlic in a food processor and pulse to chop.

2. Add the peanut butter, soy sauce, vinegar, sugar, oil, and cayenne and process until smooth and well combined. Taste and season with additional cayenne, if desired.

3. Add water, 1 tablespoon at a time, until the desired consistency is reached.

4. Serve immediately or store the sauce in a covered container in the refrigerator for up to 1 week.

Fresh and Zingy Salsa Verde

SERVES 4

▸ *SODIUM //* **6 MG**

LOW-FAT // MAKE AHEAD // QUICK

This pretty green salsa is perfect for spicing up chicken, fish, or seafood dishes. It also makes a fantastic enchilada sauce or a dip for baked tortilla chips. If you prefer a milder version, remove the seeds from the jalapeños.

2 (12-ounce) cans tomatillos, drained
1 small yellow onion, quartered
½ cup fresh cilantro
1 or 2 jalapeños
Juice of 1 lime
1 garlic clove
¼ teaspoon sugar
1 medium avocado, pitted, peeled, and diced

1. Place the tomatillos, onion, cilantro, jalapeños, lime juice, garlic, and sugar in a food processor and pulse to a chunky puree.

2. Transfer the mixture to a bowl and stir in the avocado.

3. Serve immediately or cover and refrigerate the salsa for up to 3 days.

Roasted Garlic and Rosemary Spread

SERVES 6

▸ *SODIUM //* **100 MG**

BUDGET-FRIENDLY // MAKE AHEAD

It may sound too good to be true, but this delicious spread is a snap to make and protects against heart disease, diabetes, cancer, and vampires. Seriously, garlic is one of the healthiest foods there is, possessing antibacterial, antiviral, and anti-inflammatory properties; blood-thinning and cholesterol-lowering compounds; and antioxidants that protect against disease. Roasting the garlic mellows it and brings out its natural sweetness. Use this versatile condiment as a sandwich spread, a base for salad dressings, or a sauce for roasted or grilled vegetables, meats, or fish.

1 garlic head

3 tablespoons olive oil

1 tablespoon minced fresh rosemary

¼ teaspoon freshly ground pepper

3 tablespoons fresh lemon juice

1. Preheat the oven to 400°F.

2. Slice the top ½ inch off the head of garlic so that the tops of the cloves are exposed. Place the garlic on a square of aluminum foil and drizzle 1 tablespoon of the oil over the top. Wrap up the garlic in the foil, leaving a bit of room inside for air to circulate.

3. Roast the garlic in the oven for 50 to 60 minutes, until the garlic cloves are soft and browned. Remove the garlic from the oven and let it cool.

4. Once the garlic is cool enough to handle, squeeze the cloves out of the peel and place them in a small bowl.

5. Add the rosemary and pepper and mash to a paste with a fork.

6. Stir in the lemon juice and remaining 2 tablespoons oil and mix well.

7. Serve immediately or cover and refrigerate the spread for up to 1 week.

CHAPTER NINE

Salads and Dressings

S alads may be thought of as the quintessential health food, but the reality is that many are weighed down with ingredients that are high in fat, calories, and sodium. However, done right, salads are a great way to get lots of vegetables into your daily diet.

The trick to making healthful salads that you'll actually want to eat again and again, of course, is using nutritious ingredients with lots of flavor (and not a lot of sodium). In this chapter, you'll find recipes for truly good-for-you salads that combine interesting flavors, textures, and health benefits to make them a great part of your everyday diet.

Garlic-Dijon Vinaigrette

SERVES 6

▶ *SODIUM //* **98 MG**

BUDGET-FRIENDLY // LOW-FAT // QUICK

Every home cook should have an easy but fantastic vinaigrette in his or her culinary repertoire. This one is delicious on its own, and also serves as a great base for variations. Try adding a dash of Worcestershire sauce, citrus zest, minced fresh herbs, or flavored vinegars to create your own signature dressings.

3 tablespoons water

2 tablespoons fresh lemon juice

2 tablespoons wine vinegar (red or white)

1 tablespoon Dijon mustard

1 garlic clove

½ teaspoon freshly ground pepper

3 tablespoons olive oil

1. In a food processor, combine the water, lemon juice, vinegar, mustard, garlic, and pepper and process until well combined.

2. With the processor running, add the oil in a thin stream and process until the mixture is emulsified.

3. Serve immediately or cover and refrigerate the dressing for up to 1 week. Shake or whisk before serving to re-emulsify after refrigeration.

Sesame-Ginger Dressing

SERVES 6

▶ *SODIUM //* **153 MG**
LOW-FAT // QUICK

In addition to being full of vitamins and minerals, sesame seeds, which are among the oldest of condiments used by humans, contain a special type of fiber called lignans that can help to lower cholesterol. This quick, simple dressing is lovely on a salad with mixed greens, cucumbers, and avocado or anytime you want a salad with Asian flair.

....

½ cup rice wine vinegar

¼ cup water

2 tablespoons tahini

2 tablespoons sugar

1 (2-inch) length fresh ginger, peeled and roughly chopped

1 tablespoon low-sodium soy sauce

4 teaspoons canola oil

2 teaspoons dark sesame oil

....

1. In a food processor, combine all of the ingredients and process until well combined.

2. Serve immediately or cover and refrigerate the dressing for up to 1 week.

Roasted Beet Salad with Goat Cheese

SERVES 4

▶ *SODIUM //* **286 MG**
LOW-FAT // MAKE AHEAD

With their gorgeous red color and succulent texture, roasted beets add a touch of elegance to a simple salad. Of course, they are also full of antioxidants and vitamin C, making them as healthful as they are glamorous. Serve this salad as a first course followed by a healthful steak or lamb dish for your next dinner party.

1 pound beets
1 tablespoon vinegar
1 garlic clove, minced
½ teaspoon freshly ground pepper
2 tablespoons olive oil
¼ cup fresh mint, coarsely chopped
2 ounces goat cheese, crumbled
2 tablespoons crushed roasted unsalted pistachios

1. Preheat the oven to 375°F.

2. Trim the beets and wrap them in aluminum foil. Place the foil packet on a baking sheet and bake for 60 to 70 minutes, until the beets are tender. Remove the beets from the foil and allow to cool.

3. When the beets are cool enough to handle, slip the peels off the beets and discard them. Slice the beets into thin rounds.

4. In a medium bowl, combine the vinegar, garlic, and pepper. Add the oil and whisk until combined. Add the beets and toss to coat.

5. Marinate the beets in the bowl in the refrigerator for at least 4 hours or overnight.

6. To serve, arrange the sliced beets on a platter and sprinkle with the mint, goat cheese, and pistachios.

Baby Greens Salad with Ginger Dressing

SERVES 4

▶ *SODIUM //* **225 MG**
QUICK

This simple, quick salad is full of leafy greens and other healthful veggies like radishes, and the dressing is fortified with a kick of ginger. It is perfect on its own as a light snack or served alongside a spicy Asian stir-fry.

For the dressing:

3 tablespoons minced onion

2 tablespoons rice vinegar

2 tablespoons canola oil

1½ tablespoons finely grated peeled fresh ginger

1 tablespoon ketchup

1 tablespoon low-sodium soy sauce

1 teaspoon sesame oil

For the salad:

12 ounces mixed baby greens

½ medium red bell pepper, diced

½ medium cucumber, halved lengthwise and thinly sliced

4 radishes, thinly sliced

To make the dressing:

1. In a small bowl, whisk together the onion, vinegar, canola oil, ginger, ketchup, soy sauce, and sesame oil until well combined.

To make the salad:

1. In a large salad bowl, toss together the baby greens, bell pepper, cucumber, and radishes.

2. Add the dressing and toss to coat evenly. Serve immediately.

Radicchio, Fennel, and Orange Salad with Olive Vinaigrette

SERVES 4

▶ *SODIUM //* **163 MG**
LOW-FAT // QUICK

Fennel contains a unique combination of phytonutrients that gives it strong anti-oxidant properties. Among these phytonutrients is an anti-inflammatory compound that has been shown to reduce the risk of cancer. Radicchio is a reddish-purple leafy green with a bitter bite that balances well with the anise of the fennel.

For the vinaigrette:
½ teaspoon orange zest
½ cup fresh orange juice
¼ cup apple cider vinegar
¼ cup pitted and chopped kalamata olives
1 tablespoon minced fresh oregano
1 teaspoon Dijon mustard
½ teaspoon freshly ground pepper
1 tablespoon olive oil

For the salad:
3 heads radicchio, torn into bite-size pieces
2 medium fennel bulbs, trimmed and thinly sliced
2 medium oranges (such as Valencia or navel)

To make the dressing:

1. In a small bowl, whisk together the orange zest, orange juice, vinegar, olives, oregano, mustard, and pepper. Slowly whisk in the oil.

To make the salad:

1. Toss the radicchio and fennel together in a large salad bowl.

2. Peel the oranges with a sharp knife, removing all of the white pith. Quarter the oranges, and thinly slice each quarter crosswise. Add the orange slices to the salad bowl and toss to combine.

3. Drizzle the dressing over the salad and toss to coat well. Serve immediately.

Heart-Healthful Cobb Salad

SERVES 4

▸ *SODIUM //* **390 MG**
QUICK

Traditional Cobb salad is loaded with sodium—from bacon, blue cheese, and salty dressing. Here we've reduced the sodium level significantly, without sacrificing any of the crunchy, salty, tangy flavor and texture that we love in a Cobb salad. Turkey bacon subs for saltier (and fattier) pork bacon, and the blue cheese is right in the dressing, allowing this recipe to omit salt in the dressing while ensuring that the rich, tangy blue cheese flavor is well distributed throughout the salad.

For the dressing:
¼ cup water
3 tablespoons white wine vinegar
1 tablespoon minced shallot
1 teaspoon Dijon mustard
½ teaspoon freshly ground pepper
¼ cup crumbled blue cheese

For the salad:
1 large head romaine lettuce, chopped
8 ounces cooked chicken breast, diced or shredded
2 eggs, hard-boiled, peeled, and chopped
2 medium tomatoes, diced
1 large cucumber, seeded and sliced
½ avocado, diced
2 slices cooked turkey bacon, crumbled

To make the dressing:

1. Whisk together the water, vinegar, shallot, mustard, and pepper in a small bowl until well combined. Add the cheese and stir to mix well.

To make the salad:

1. Place the lettuce in a large mixing bowl and drizzle with half of the dressing. Toss to coat.

2. Arrange the lettuce on 4 serving plates. Top with the chicken, eggs, tomatoes, cucumber, avocado, and bacon, arranging each ingredient in a line.

3. Drizzle the remaining dressing over the salads and serve immediately.

Smoked Eggplant Salad with Tomato Vinaigrette

SERVES 4

▸ *SODIUM //* **299 MG**
LOW-FAT

Eggplant is prized for its deep purple color, but more important, it contains phyto-nutrients, which are high in antioxidants. Low in calories and full of fiber, eggplants also contain phytonutrients that improve blood circulation and lower cholesterol. Plus, it's delicious.

1 large eggplant
½ teaspoon salt
Cooking spray
2 tablespoons sherry vinegar
1 medium tomato, quartered
1 garlic clove
1½ teaspoons smoked paprika
¼ cup olive oil
4 cups mixed baby lettuces

1. Preheat a barbecue, gas grill, or grill pan to medium heat.

2. Line a large baking sheet with a double layer of paper towels.

3. Slice the eggplant into ¼-inch-thick rounds. Sprinkle both sides with salt and then lay them on the prepared baking sheet. Let sit for 10 minutes.

4. Dry the eggplant slices, blotting them with paper towels, and spray them lightly with the cooking spray. Cook the eggplant slices in a single layer on the grill for 5 to 6 minutes per side, until they are soft and cooked through with nice grill marks.

5. To make the dressing, in a food processor or blender, combine the vinegar, tomato, garlic, and paprika and process until smooth. Whisk in the oil.

6. In a medium mixing bowl, toss the lettuce with half of the vinaigrette.

7. Arrange the eggplant slices on 4 salad plates and spoon the remaining vinaigrette over them, dividing it equally. Put a handful of the dressed lettuce on top of each serving of eggplant. Serve immediately.

Baby Blues Salad

SERVES 4

▶ *SODIUM //* **298 MG**
QUICK

Blueberries have one of the highest antioxidant levels of any food, making them a true super food, fighting disease while making every dish they find themselves in more delicious. Here they are combined with baby lettuces, blue cheese, and almonds for an eye-catching salad with an unusual and surprisingly delicious combination of flavors.

For the dressing:
2 tablespoons balsamic vinegar
1½ tablespoons water
1 teaspoon Dijon mustard
½ teaspoon freshly ground pepper
3 tablespoons olive oil

For the salad:
8 cups mixed baby lettuce, torn into bite-size pieces
2 cups fresh blueberries
½ cup crumbled blue cheese
¼ cup sliced almonds

To make the dressing:

1. In a small bowl, whisk together the vinegar, water, mustard, and pepper until well combined.

2. Slowly add the oil in a thin stream while continuing to whisk until the mixture is emulsified.

To make the salad:

1. Place the lettuce in a large salad bowl. Add the blueberries and toss to combine. Add the dressing and toss to coat.

2. Sprinkle the cheese and almonds over the top and serve immediately.

Caesar Salad Revamp

SERVES 6

▶ *SODIUM* // **343 MG**
QUICK

Classic Caesar salads are loaded with sodium. This recipe reduces the salt significantly without eliminating the classic flavors—anchovies, Worcestershire sauce, lemon, and Parmesan cheese—that you expect from a good Caesar. Romaine lettuce is an often overlooked nutrition powerhouse. Its high doses of vitamin C, beta-carotene, folic acid, potassium, and fiber combine to reduce the risk of heart disease, including high blood pressure, heart attack, and stroke. In short, a Caesar a day might just keep the heart doctor away.

For the croutons:
4 slices sourdough bread, cubed
1 tablespoon unsalted butter, melted
¾ teaspoon garlic powder

For the dressing:
1 egg yolk
3 tablespoons fresh lemon juice
1 tablespoon red wine vinegar
2 garlic cloves, minced
1½ teaspoons anchovy paste
1 teaspoon Worcestershire sauce
½ teaspoon freshly ground pepper
⅓ cup olive oil

For the salad:
1 head romaine lettuce, torn into bite-size pieces
2 tablespoons grated Parmesan cheese, for garnish

continued ▶

To make the croutons:

1. Preheat the oven to 350°F.

2. On a large baking sheet, toss together the bread, butter, and garlic powder until the bread is well coated. Bake the bread in the oven for 18 to 20 minutes, turning once, until lightly browned and crisp.

3. Remove the croutons from the oven and let them cool to room temperature.

To make the dressing:

1. Whisk together the egg yolk, lemon juice, vinegar, garlic, anchovy paste, Worcestershire sauce, and pepper until well combined.

2. Slowly whisk in the oil until the mixture is emulsified.

To make the salad:

1. Place the lettuce in a large salad bowl and toss with the dressing until everything is well coated.

2. Serve immediately, garnished with the croutons and Parmesan cheese.

Warm Sweet Potato Salad with Balsamic Vinaigrette

SERVES 6

SODIUM // **24 MG**
LOW-FAT // QUICK

This quick and easy salad is a twist on the classic warm potato salad. Replacing white potatoes with sweet potatoes boosts the nutritional content and makes it stunning to look at, too. Serve this at your next barbecue and you may never go back to the old mayo-and-white-potato version.

2 pounds sweet potatoes, peeled and cut into 1-inch cubes
3 tablespoons balsamic vinegar
1 tablespoon cider vinegar
1 teaspoon Dijon mustard
½ teaspoon honey
¼ cup olive oil
1 small stalk celery, very finely diced
1 tablespoon minced shallots
2 teaspoons chopped fresh chives
2 teaspoons chopped fresh parsley
½ teaspoon freshly ground pepper

1. Place the potatoes in a large pot and cover with about 3 inches of water. Bring the water to a boil over high heat, and then reduce the heat to medium-low and simmer for about 15 minutes, until the potatoes are tender. Drain and transfer the potatoes to a large salad bowl.

2. While the potatoes are simmering, make the dressing. In a small bowl, whisk together the vinegars, mustard, and honey until well combined.

3. Add the oil while whisking constantly until the mixture is emulsified.

4. Stir in the celery, shallots, chives, parsley, and pepper.

5. Toss the dressing with the warm potatoes and serve immediately.

CHAPTER TEN

Soups, Chilies, and Stews

Soups, chilies, and stews are welcome comfort foods on rainy days, cold winter nights, or whenever you are feeling a bit under the weather. Unfortunately, most store-bought varieties and many recipes for homemade soups and stews are full of unwanted sodium.

This chapter includes recipes for both hearty and light soups, chilies, and stews that will warm you up without all that added sodium (or excessive fat, either). Whether you're in the mood for vegetarian soup, hearty chili, rich beef stew, simple tomato soup, or elegant seafood bouillabaisse, this chapter has got you covered.

Roasted Tomato Soup with Mint

SERVES 4

▶ *SODIUM //* **150 MG**

BUDGET-FRIENDLY // LOW-FAT // MAKE AHEAD

This soup is amazingly easy to make and surprisingly delicious. Loaded with disease-fighting lycopene and vitamin C, it is also impressively healthful. If you're craving this soup when tomatoes aren't in season, you can substitute canned fire-roasted tomatoes (look for a no-salt-added variety), adding them to the food processor along with the roasted onions and garlic.

3 pounds plum tomatoes, halved lengthwise
1 large yellow onion, chopped
4 garlic cloves, minced
2 tablespoons olive oil
1 teaspoon freshly ground pepper
6 cups low-sodium chicken or vegetable broth
Juice of 1 lemon
1 cup chopped fresh mint

1. Preheat the oven to 400°F.

2. On a large baking sheet, toss the tomatoes, onion, and garlic with the oil and pepper. Spread the tomatoes out in a single layer, cut side up, and roast them in the oven until they are very soft, about 45 minutes.

3. Transfer the vegetables to a food processor or blender and puree until smooth.

4. Pour the puree into a large stockpot, add the broth, and bring to a boil over medium-high heat. Stir in the lemon juice and simmer until heated through.

5. Stir in the mint and serve immediately. This soup will keep, covered, in the refrigerator for up to 1 week or in the freezer for up to 3 months.

Green Soup with Goat Cheese

SERVES 4

▶ *SODIUM //* **270 MG**

MAKE AHEAD // QUICK

Calorie for calorie, dark leafy greens represent the most concentrated sources of nutrients you can find, including vitamins like B, C, E, and K; minerals like iron and magnesium; and phytonutrients like beta-carotene. The luscious green hue of this soup is proof of just how good it is for you, packed as it is with spinach (one of the most nutrient-dense greens), watercress, and sorrel. Goat cheese adds rich creaminess, while the watercress and sorrel provide a peppery kick and lemony tang. If you can't find sorrel, simply use more spinach and stir in a couple of tablespoons of lemon juice just before serving.

....

1 tablespoon plus 1 teaspoon extra-virgin olive oil

2 leeks, green and light green parts, thinly sliced

2 tablespoons sherry

4 cups low-sodium vegetable broth

2 cups water

1 potato, peeled and diced

1 pound spinach leaves, tough stems trimmed and discarded

2 cups watercress

2 cups sorrel

¼ teaspoon cayenne pepper

½ cup crumbled goat cheese, plus more for garnish

2 tablespoons unsalted butter

Freshly ground pepper

....

1. Heat the oil in a large stockpot over medium-high heat. Add the leeks and cook, stirring frequently, until soft, about 5 minutes.

2. Add the sherry and cook, stirring, until the liquid has evaporated.

continued ▶

3. Add the broth, water, and diced potato and bring to a boil. Reduce the heat to low and simmer, uncovered, for about 15 minutes, until the potato pieces are tender.

4. Stir in the spinach, watercress, sorrel, and cayenne. Cook, covered, for about 5 minutes, until the spinach is tender.

5. Remove the pot from the heat, add the goat cheese and butter, and stir until they are well incorporated.

6. Using an immersion blender or in batches in a blender, puree the soup until smooth. Reheat if needed.

7. Serve immediately, garnished with a bit of crumbled goat cheese and a generous sprinkling of pepper. The soup will keep for up to 3 days in the refrigerator.

Curried Sweet Potato Soup

SERVES 4

▸ *SODIUM* // **326 MG**

LOW-FAT // MAKE AHEAD // QUICK

Sweet potatoes are lauded by nutritionists as one of the most nutrient-dense vegetables. They are loaded with vitamins B_6, C, and D as well as heart-healthful minerals like magnesium and potassium. Here we've spiced them up with curry powder and fresh ginger for a satisfying soup that's perfect for lunch or dinner.

1 tablespoon olive oil

1 medium onion, chopped

3 cups water

1½ cups low-sodium vegetable or chicken broth

2 large sweet potatoes, peeled and diced

2 large carrots, sliced

1 tablespoon minced peeled fresh ginger

1 tablespoon curry powder

Freshly ground pepper

1. Heat the oil in a large stockpot over medium-high heat. Add the onion and cook, stirring frequently, until soft, about 5 minutes.

2. Add the the water, broth, sweet potatoes, carrots, ginger, and curry powder. Bring to a boil, reduce the heat to medium-low, and simmer, uncovered, until the vegetables are tender, about 20 minutes.

3. Using an immersion blender or in batches in a blender, puree the mixture. If the soup is too thick, add a bit more broth.

4. Reheat the soup, if needed. Season with the pepper and serve immediately. The soup will keep in the refrigerator for up to 1 week or in the freezer for up to 3 months.

Smoky Red Lentil Soup

SERVES 4

▶ *SODIUM //* **153 MG**

BUDGET-FRIENDLY // LOW-FAT // MAKE AHEAD // QUICK

Red lentils make a beautifully red-hued soup. With the addition of paprika and tur-meric, this version is particularly stunning. Quick cooking, full of fiber, and delicious, lentils are an excellent and inexpensive source of vegetarian protein. This spicy soup gets better with time, so make it a day or two ahead if you are able, or make a double batch and eat leftovers all week.

1 tablespoon olive oil
1 medium onion, diced
2 garlic cloves, minced
2 teaspoons ground cumin
2 teaspoons smoked paprika
1 teaspoon sweet paprika
1 teaspoon ground turmeric
¼ teaspoon ground cinnamon
2 medium carrots, sliced
7 cups low-sodium vegetable broth
1½ cups dry red lentils
1 (14-ounce) can no-salt-added diced tomatoes, with juice
Juice of 1 lemon
Lemon wedges, for garnish
¼ cup minced fresh parsley, for garnish

1. Heat the oil in a large stockpot over medium-high heat. Add the onions and garlic and sauté, stirring frequently, until the onions have softened, about 5 minutes.

2. Stir in the cumin, smoked and sweet paprika, turmeric, and cinnamon and cook, stirring, for 1 minute.

3. Add the carrots, broth and lentils. Bring the liquid to a boil, reduce the heat to medium-low, and simmer, uncovered, until the lentils are soft, 30 to 35 minutes.

4. Add the tomatoes along with their juice and cook for 10 minutes more.

5. Just before serving, stir in the lemon juice.

6. Serve hot, garnished with lemon wedges and a generous sprinkling of parsley.

Creamy Broccoli-Cheese Soup

SERVES 4

▶ *SODIUM //* **344 MG**
QUICK

We don't have to tell you how great broccoli is for you, but did you know that cooking broccoli increases its ability to lower cholesterol? This lightened-up version of a classic soup uses the stems and florets and gives you all the flavor you expect from a broccoli-cheese soup with far less fat and calories, not to mention sodium.

1 tablespoon olive oil
1 head broccoli, stems peeled and chopped, florets separated
1 medium onion, diced
8 ounces new potatoes, diced
¼ cup all-purpose flour
3½ cups low-sodium chicken or vegetable broth
¼ teaspoon freshly grated nutmeg
1 cup grated reduced-fat cheddar cheese
1 (12-ounce) can fat-free evaporated milk
1 teaspoon Worcestershire sauce
½ teaspoon freshly ground pepper
2 green onions, thinly sliced

1. Heat the oil in a large stockpot over medium heat. Add the broccoli stems, onion, and potatoes. Cook stirring frequently, until the vegetables begin to soften, about 10 minutes.

2. Sprinkle the flour into the pot and cook, stirring constantly, until it begins to give off a slightly nutty aroma, about 2 minutes.

3. Add the broth and bring it to a boil. Reduce the heat to medium-low and cook, stirring occasionally, for about 15 minutes, until the vegetables are soft. Add the broccoli florets and cook about 5 minutes more, until the florets are tender.

4. Sprinkle in the nutmeg and stir to combine.

5. Remove the pot from the heat and stir in the cheese, milk, Worcestershire sauce, and pepper.

6. Puree the soup using an immersion blender or in batches in a traditional blender or food processor.

7. Serve immediately, garnished with the green onions.

Lemony Chicken Noodle Soup

SERVES 4

▸ *SODIUM //* **114 MG**

BUDGET-FRIENDLY // LOW-FAT // MAKE AHEAD

The ultimate comfort food, chicken noodle soup is the perfect meal whether you need to feed a cold or are just craving a little bit of feel-good in a bowl. Once you try this lemony, veggie-filled version, you'll swear off the canned stuff—which is loaded with sodium—for good.

6 cups low-sodium chicken broth

2 cups water

1⅓ cups chopped carrot

1¼ cups chopped onion

1 cup chopped celery

1 pound cooked chicken breast, shredded or diced

8 ounces dried egg noodles, cooked according to package directions

¼ cup chopped fresh flat-leaf parsley

Zest and juice of 1 lemon

1. In a large stockpot over medium-high heat, combine the broth, water, carrot, onion, and celery and bring to a boil. Reduce the heat to medium-low and simmer, covered, until the vegetables are tender, about 20 minutes.

2. Add the chicken and noodles and simmer until heated through, about 3 minutes.

3. Stir in the parsley, lemon zest, and lemon juice. Serve immediately.

White Bean and Greens Soup with Sausage

SERVES 6

▸ *SODIUM* // **480 MG**

MAKE AHEAD // *QUICK*

White beans are another excellent source of protein that is full of fiber and anti-oxidants. A hefty serving of super-healthful kale adds even more essential vitamins, minerals, fiber, and antioxidants. While cured meats are usually a no-no for those on low-sodium diets, this soup gets a big dose of meaty flavor from a small amount of flavorful smoked sausage. With a loaf of crusty bread and a crisp green salad, this hearty soup makes a perfect meal for a cold evening.

2 tablespoons olive oil

1 medium onion, diced

2 garlic cloves, minced

2 stalks celery, sliced

2 medium carrots, sliced

6 ounces Spanish-style chorizo or andouille sausage, diced

1 bunch kale, chopped

4 cups low-sodium chicken broth

1 (14-ounce) can no-salt-added diced tomatoes, with juice

1 (15-ounce) can white beans, such as cannellini or great northern, drained and rinsed

½ teaspoon freshly ground pepper

1. Heat the oil in a large stockpot over medium-high heat. Add the onion and garlic and cook, stirring frequently, until the onions are soft, about 5 minutes.

2. Add the celery, carrots, and sausage and cook, stirring occasionally, for 3 minutes more. Stir in the kale.

3. Add the broth, tomatoes with their juice, beans, and pepper and bring to a boil. Reduce the heat to medium-low and simmer, covered, for 15 to 20 minutes, until the vegetables are soft. Serve immediately.

Spicy Chicken-Chipotle Tortilla Soup

SERVES 4

▶ *SODIUM //* **340 MG**
LOW-FAT // QUICK

This is classic comfort food with a kick—a healthful chicken soup flavored with a bit of turkey bacon, thickened with crushed tortilla chips, and spiced with ground chipotle chili powder and cumin. A squeeze of lime juice and sprinkling of fresh cilantro are the perfect finishing touches.

2 slices turkey bacon
1 tablespoon olive oil
1 small yellow onion, diced
2 garlic cloves, minced
¾ pound chicken breast, diced
1 teaspoon chipotle chili powder
1 teaspoon ground cumin
3 cups low-sodium chicken broth
1 cup water
1 (14-ounce) can no-salt-added crushed tomatoes, with juice
Juice of 1 lime
1 cup crushed low-sodium baked tortilla chips
¼ cup chopped fresh cilantro, for garnish

1. In a large stockpot over medium-high heat, cook the turkey bacon until crisp. Drain the bacon on paper towels, crumble, and set aside.

2. In the same stockpot, heat the oil over medium-high heat. Add the onion and garlic and cook, stirring, until the onion is soft, about 5 minutes.

3. Add the chicken and cook, stirring, for about 2 minutes, until the chicken is opaque.

4. Add the chili powder and cumin and cook for about 30 seconds more.

5. Add the broth, water, tomatoes with their juice, and cooked turkey bacon and bring to a boil. Reduce the heat to medium, cover, and cook for about 5 minutes. Stir in the lime juice.

6. To serve, divide the crushed tortilla chips among 4 soup bowls, ladle the soup over the top, and garnish with cilantro.

Vietnamese Beef Noodle Soup with Fresh Herbs

SERVES 4

▸ *SODIUM //* **478 MG**
LOW-FAT // QUICK

This classic soup, called pho *in Vietnam, is the country's quintessential comfort food. Time-tested recipes for the flavorful broth are passed down from generation to generation. Here we start with low-sodium beef broth and give it a quick simmer with aromatic spices to get that classic flavor. This simple soup comes alive when the garnishes of fresh herbs, chilies, bean sprouts, and lime juice are added. And the best part is that each diner gets to customize his or her own bowl.*

For the soup:

6 cups low-sodium beef broth

2 cups water

1 large onion, thinly sliced

5 (½-inch-thick) slices peeled fresh ginger

1 tablespoon fish sauce

3 large garlic cloves, halved

2 star anise pods

1 teaspoon whole cloves

1 pound flank steak, trimmed, very thinly sliced crosswise

8 ounces bean thread noodles, cooked according to package directions

For the garnishes:

1½ cups bean sprouts

1 cup fresh mint

1 cup fresh basil

1 cup fresh cilantro

2 limes, cut into wedges

3 red or green jalapeños, thinly sliced

3 green onions, thinly sliced

To make the soup:

1. In a large stockpot over medium-high heat, combine the broth, water, onion, ginger, fish sauce, garlic, star anise, and cloves and bring to a boil. Reduce the heat to medium-low, cover, and simmer for about 20 minutes.

2. Strain the broth through a fine-mesh sieve into a large bowl. Discard the solids.

3. Return the broth to the pot and bring it back up to a boil. Remove from the heat and immediately add the steak slices.

To prepare the garnishes:

1. Arrange the garnishes on a platter.

2. Divide the noodles among 4 soup bowls. Ladle the hot soup over the noodles, dividing the meat evenly among the bowls.

3. Serve immediately with the platter of garnishes, instructing guests to garnish their soup as desired.

Cherry Tomato and Corn Chowder

SERVES 4

▶ *SODIUM //* **313 MG**

BUDGET-FRIENDLY // LOW-FAT // QUICK

Traditional chowders are usually loaded with calories, fat, and sodium. This quick version uses healthful substitutions—turkey bacon, low-fat milk, and low-sodium broth—to keep it healthful. Pureeing most of the corn kernels along with low-fat milk makes the chowder thick and satisfying, while the tomatoes give it unmistakable summer flavor and a pretty pop of color. For a vegetarian version, simply leave out the bacon.

....

1 tablespoon olive oil
1 medium onion, diced
2 stalks celery, diced
2 garlic cloves, minced
1 pint small cherry tomatoes, halved
2½ cups frozen corn kernels, thawed
2 cups low-fat milk
1 teaspoon chopped fresh thyme
¼ teaspoon freshly ground pepper
1 cup low-sodium vegetable or chicken broth
3 green onions, thinly sliced, for garnish
2 slices turkey bacon, cooked and crumbled, for garnish (optional)

....

1. Heat the oil in a large stockpot over medium-high heat. Add the onion, celery, and garlic and cook, stirring, until the onion is soft, about 5 minutes.

2. Add the tomatoes and cook for another 2 to 3 minutes, until the tomatoes just begin to break down.

3. Place 1½ cups of the corn, 1 cup of the milk, the thyme, and the pepper in a blender or food processor and process until smooth.

4. Transfer the pureed mixture to the stockpot and bring to a simmer.

5. Add the remaining 1 cup of corn and 1 cup of milk to the pot along with the broth. Stir well and cook over medium heat for about 5 minutes until heated through.

6. Serve hot, garnished with the green onions and bacon.

Vegetarian Quinoa Chili

SERVES 6

▸ *SODIUM //* **452 MG**

BUDGET-FRIENDLY // LOW-FAT

Quinoa is the current darling of the health food world, and for good reason. This great-tasting whole grain is full of protein and fiber, low in fat, and has a low glycemic index. It's an interesting alternative for rice or potatoes, and a great gluten-free substitute for pasta or couscous. Here it is paired with jalapeños and beans in a flavorful vegetarian chili.

½ cup quinoa, rinsed

1 tablespoon olive oil

1 small onion, chopped

2 garlic cloves, minced

2 jalapeños, seeded and diced

1 large carrot, diced

2 stalks celery, diced

1 yellow or orange bell pepper, seeded and diced

2 tablespoons chili powder

1 tablespoon ground cumin

2 (15-ounce) cans pinto beans, drained and rinsed

1 (28-ounce) can no-salt-added diced tomatoes, drained

1 (15-ounce) can low-sodium tomato sauce

1. Cook the quinoa according to the package directions.

2. Heat the oil in a large stockpot set over medium-high heat. Add the onion and garlic and cook, stirring frequently, until the onion is soft, about 5 minutes.

3. Add the jalapeños, carrot, celery, and bell pepper and cook, stirring occasionally, for about 10 minutes, until the vegetables are tender.

4. Stir in the chili powder and cumin and cook about 30 seconds more.

5. Add the beans, tomatoes, tomato sauce, and cooked quinoa. Reduce the heat to medium-low, cover, and simmer for about 30 minutes.

6. Serve hot, garnished with diced avocados, minced red onion, salsa, sour cream, or baked tortilla chips, if desired.

Bouillabaisse

SERVES 4

▶ *SODIUM //* **390 MG** *(403 MG WITH THE AIOLI)*
LOW-FAT // QUICK

Low-fat, low-calorie, and low-sodium halibut is loaded with protein and nutrients— magnesium, vitamins B_6 and B_{12}, and omega-3 fatty acids, among others. This classic French seafood stew brings them together in a rich tomato-based broth with a hint of orange. Serve it with crusty bread for soaking up the sauce, if desired.

For the stew:
1 tablespoon extra-virgin olive oil
2 garlic cloves, minced
1 medium shallot, diced
¾ cup low-sodium fish or chicken broth
¾ cup dry white wine
1 (14-ounce) can no-salt-added diced tomatoes, drained
2 teaspoons fresh thyme, or ¾ teaspoon dried thyme
2 teaspoons orange zest
1 teaspoon smoked paprika
½ teaspoon red pepper flakes
½ teaspoon saffron threads, crushed
12 ounces skinless halibut fillets, cut into 1-inch pieces
¼ cup minced fresh flat-leaf parsley, for garnish

For the aioli (optional):
¼ cup reduced-fat mayonnaise
1 garlic clove, minced
2 teaspoons fresh lemon juice

To make the stew:

1. Heat the oil in a large skillet or Dutch oven over medium-high heat. Add the garlic and shallot and cook, stirring, until the shallot is soft, about 5 minutes.

2. Add the broth and wine and simmer for 2 minutes more.

3. Add the tomatoes, thyme, orange zest, smoked paprika, red pepper flakes, and saffron and simmer for 2 minutes more.

4. Add the fish, cover, and continue to simmer until the fish is cooked through, about 6 minutes.

To make the aioli (if using):

1. In a small bowl, stir together the mayonnaise, garlic, and lemon juice until well combined.

2. Ladle the stew into shallow bowls, and garnish with the parsley and a dollop of aioli, if using. Serve immediately.

White Chicken Chili

SERVES 4

▶ *SODIUM //* **302 MG**

BUDGET-FRIENDLY // MAKE AHEAD // QUICK

White chili offers all the hearty flavors of a classic chili but with many fewer calories and fat grams. Garnish this spicy version with diced avocado, fresh salsa, low-fat sour cream, shredded low-sodium cheese, or baked tortilla chips as desired. Chili is one of those dishes that gets better with time. Make a double batch and store the extra in a sealed container in the refrigerator for up to three days or in the freezer for up to three months.

1 tablespoon canola oil

1 onion, chopped

3 garlic cloves, minced

1 to 3 jalapeños, seeded and diced

2 (4-ounce) cans mild diced green chilies

2 teaspoons ground cumin

1½ teaspoons ground coriander

1 teaspoon chili powder

1 teaspoon dried oregano

¼ to ½ teaspoon cayenne pepper

2 (14-ounce) cans low-sodium chicken broth

3 cups chopped cooked chicken breast

3 (15-ounce) cans white beans

¼ cup chopped fresh cilantro, for garnish

1. Heat the oil in a large stockpot over medium heat. Add the onion and garlic and cook, stirring frequently, until the onion is soft, about 5 minutes.

2. Add the jalapeño(s), green chilies, cumin, coriander, chili powder, oregano, and cayenne. Cook, stirring frequently, for 2 to 3 minutes, until the chilies begin to soften.

3. Add the broth, chicken, and beans and bring to a boil over medium-high heat. Reduce the heat to medium-low and simmer, uncovered, stirring occasionally, for about 15 minutes.

4. Serve hot, garnished with the cilantro.

Chicken and Shrimp Gumbo

SERVES 4

▶ *SODIUM* // **488 MG**

QUICK

Cajun food is known for its intense flavors and indulgent amounts of fat. This version of the classic Cajun stew is significantly lighter than most, with much less sodium. But don't worry; it's still full of delicious spice and hearty Cajun flavor.

....

2 tablespoons canola oil

¼ cup all-purpose flour

1 medium onion, diced

1 green bell pepper, seeded and diced

2 stalks celery, diced

3 garlic cloves, minced

1 tablespoon minced fresh thyme, or 1 teaspoon dried thyme

¼ to ½ teaspoon cayenne pepper

½ cup dry white wine

1 (14-ounce) can no-salt-added diced tomatoes, with juice

2 cups water

1 (10-ounce) package frozen sliced okra

4 ounces smoked andouille sausage, diced

1 pound medium shrimp, peeled and deveined

1½ pounds cooked chicken breast, diced

¼ cup minced fresh flat-leaf parsley, for garnish

....

1. Heat the oil in a large stockpot or Dutch oven over medium-high heat. Add the flour and cook, whisking constantly, until the mixture turns chestnut brown and gives off a nutty aroma, about 5 minutes.

continued ▶

2. Add the onion, bell pepper, celery, and garlic and cook, stirring occasionally, until the onions are soft, about 5 minutes.

3. Add the thyme and cayenne and cook for 1 minute more.

4. Stir in the wine and bring to a boil, stirring occasionally.

5. Add the tomatoes with their juice, water, and okra and simmer, uncovered, for about 15 minutes.

6. Add the sausage and shrimp, and simmer for about 5 minutes more.

7. Stir in the cooked chicken and continue to simmer, stirring occasionally, until the chicken is heated through and the shrimp is opaque.

8. Serve hot, garnished with the parsley.

Italian Chicken Stew with Artichokes and Olives

SERVES 6

▶ *SODIUM //* **438 MG**
LOW-FAT // MAKE AHEAD

Olive oil may get all the attention from the healthful nutrition world, but olives them-selves provide many of the same beneficial nutrients, including healthful fats and disease-fighting antioxidants. Here they're paired with artichokes, which contain more antioxidants than any other vegetable, for a super-healthful stew that's also super-delicious.

....

1½ pounds boneless, skinless chicken breast, cut into bite-size pieces
1½ teaspoons freshly ground pepper
2 tablespoons all-purpose flour
2 tablespoons olive oil
2 large garlic cloves, minced
2 teaspoons capers, drained and minced
Zest of 1 lemon
½ cup dry white wine
1¾ cups low-sodium chicken broth
1 pound Yukon Gold potatoes, scrubbed and cut into ¾-inch cubes
1 (8-ounce) package frozen artichoke hearts, thawed and halved or quartered
Juice of 1 lemon
1 cup finely chopped fresh flat-leaf parsley, plus additional for garnish
¾ cup pitted medium green olives, quartered

....

1. In a large bowl, season the chicken with the pepper and toss with the flour to coat.

2. Heat the oil in a Dutch oven or large stockpot over medium-high heat. Add the chicken and cook, turning frequently, until browned on all sides, about 5 minutes total. Transfer the chicken to a bowl.

continued ▶

3. Reduce the heat to medium. Add the garlic, capers, and lemon zest and cook, stirring, for about 30 seconds.

4. Add the wine and cook, stirring and scraping up the browned bits from the bottom of the pan, for about 2 minutes, until the liquid is reduced by about half.

5. Return the cooked chicken to the pot along with the broth and potatoes. Reduce the heat to medium-low, cover, and simmer for 10 minutes.

6. Add the artichokes and continue to cook, covered, until the potatoes are tender, about 10 minutes more.

7. Add the lemon juice, parsley, and olives and stir well.

8. Serve hot, garnished with additional parsley.

Pork and Apple Stew

SERVES 4

▶ *SODIUM //* **350 MG**

MAKE AHEAD // QUICK

An apple a day keeps the doctor away, right? This old adage might actually be true since apples have lots of disease-fighting antioxidants. Here we've paired them with pork and flavorful turkey bacon for a satisfying stew with classic flavors. It's simple and quick to prepare and makes for great leftovers, too.

....

2 tablespoons canola oil

1 medium onion, diced

2 slices turkey bacon

1½ pounds boneless pork shoulder, cut into thin strips

2 large green apples, such as Granny Smith, unpeeled and
    cut into ¾-inch chunks

¾ pound small new potatoes

1 (16-ounce) package shredded green cabbage

2 cups low-sodium chicken broth

1 cup apple juice

2 tablespoons Dijon mustard

½ teaspoon freshly ground pepper

1 tablespoon white wine vinegar

1 tablespoon fresh thyme leaves, for garnish

....

1. Heat the oil in a Dutch oven or large stockpot over medium-high heat. Add the onions and bacon and cook, stirring, until the onions begin to soften and the bacon begins to brown, about 5 minutes.

2. Add the pork and cook, stirring occasionally, until the meat is browned on all sides, about 5 minutes. Transfer the mixture to a bowl.

3. Add the apples, potatoes, cabbage, broth, apple juice, mustard, and pepper to the pot and bring to a boil. Reduce the heat to medium-low and stir in the pork, onions, bacon, and vinegar. Simmer, uncovered, for about 15 minutes.

4. Serve hot, garnished with the thyme.

Mexican Pork Stew with Black Beans and Tomatillos

SERVES 6

▶ *SODIUM //* **108 MG**
LOW-FAT // MAKE AHEAD

This spicy stew may take a while to cook, but it couldn't be easier. Tomatillos, common in Mexican cooking, look like small green tomatoes covered with a papery skin. They have a tart, lemony flavor that pairs perfectly with meaty pork and spicy chilies. Look for canned tomatillos in the international foods aisle of your supermarket or at specialty Latin markets. This stew gets better with time, so make it a day or two ahead if you can, or store it in the freezer for up to three months.

1 tablespoon canola oil

1½ pounds pork tenderloin, cut into 1-inch cubes

½ teaspoon freshly ground pepper

2 medium onions, diced

4 garlic cloves, minced

2 jalapeños, seeded and diced

2 teaspoons ground cumin

2 teaspoons chili powder

1 teaspoon dried oregano

1 (28-ounce) can tomatillos, drained and diced

1 (28-ounce) can no-salt-added diced tomatoes, drained

1½ cups dark Mexican beer

1½ cups fresh orange juice

1 (15-ounce) can black beans, drained and rinsed

½ cup chopped fresh cilantro leaves, plus more for garnish

Juice of 1 lime

1. Heat the oil in a Dutch oven or large stockpot over medium-high heat. Sprinkle the pork with the pepper and add it to the pot (you may have to brown the pork in two batches to avoid crowding the stockpot). Cook, turning frequently, until the meat is browned on all sides. Transfer the meat to a large bowl.

2. Add the onions and garlic to the stockpot and cook, stirring frequently, until the onion has softened, about 5 minutes.

3. Add the jalapeños, cumin, chili powder, and oregano and cook, stirring, for 1 minute more.

4. Add the tomatillos, tomatoes, beer, and orange juice and bring to a boil. Reduce the heat to low and simmer, uncovered, for about 10 minutes.

5. Return the pork to the pot and simmer, covered, for about 2 hours, until the pork is very tender.

6. Add the beans and cilantro and cook for about 10 minutes more, until the beans are heated through.

7. Just before serving, stir in the lime juice. Serve hot, garnished with additional cilantro.

Beef and Stout Stew

SERVES 6

▶ *SODIUM //* **111 MG**

MAKE AHEAD

Serve this classic Irish stew for St. Patrick's Day, or anytime you are craving a satisfyingly rich bowl of meat stew. Beef, unfairly maligned by dieters, provides lots of protein and iron. And if you choose lean stew meat, the dish is surprisingly low in fat.

1½ pounds lean stew beef, trimmed and cut into 1-inch chunks
3 tablespoons olive oil
½ teaspoon freshly ground pepper
2 tablespoons all-purpose flour
2 large onions, diced
2 garlic cloves, minced
2 tablespoons tomato paste
1 cup stout beer
1 cup low-sodium beef broth
2 large carrots, sliced
2 teaspoons chopped fresh thyme
¼ cup minced fresh flat-leaf parsley, for garnish

1. Preheat the oven to 325°F.

2. In a large mixing bowl, combine the beef and 1 tablespoon of the oil. Sprinkle with the pepper and then add the flour and toss until the meat is well coated.

3. Heat the remaining 2 tablespoons of oil in a large Dutch oven. Add the meat and cook, turning frequently, until browned on all sides.

4. Add the onions, garlic, and tomato paste and cook, stirring frequently, for 2 to 3 minutes.

5. Add ½ cup of the stout to the pot to deglaze; stir and scrape up the browned bits from the bottom of the pan while bringing to a boil. Add the remaining ½ cup stout along with the broth, carrots, and thyme.

6. Cover and bake in the oven for 2 to 3 hours, until the meat is very tender.

7. Serve hot, garnished with the parsley, or over mashed potatoes, if desired.

Chinese-Style Beef and Vegetable Hot Pot

SERVES 6

▶ *SODIUM //* **445 MG**
LOW-FAT // MAKE AHEAD

This dish is the Chinese version of meat-and-potatoes comfort food. Flavored with soy sauce, ginger, and chili paste, it will warm you up on a cold winter's night. Between the beef and the spinach, you'll get plenty of iron, and the carrots, turnips, and potatoes deliver essential vitamins, minerals, and disease-fighting antioxidants. Believe it or not, using lean beef stew meat makes the dish low in fat.

1 tablespoon canola oil

1½ pounds lean beef stew meat, cut into 1-inch pieces

2 medium shallots, diced

2 tablespoons minced peeled fresh ginger

4 garlic cloves, minced

1 cup low-sodium beef broth

2¾ cups water

3 tablespoons Chinese cooking wine or dry sherry

2 tablespoons low-sodium soy sauce

1 tablespoon brown sugar

2 teaspoons chili paste

2 cinnamon sticks

1 star anise pod

2 large carrots, sliced

1 large turnip, diced

1 large potato, peeled and diced

1 tablespoon cornstarch, mixed with 1 tablespoon water

8 cups spinach (about ½ pound)

3 green onions, thinly sliced, for garnish

1. Heat the oil in a Dutch oven or large stockpot over medium-high heat. Add the beef and cook, turning frequently, until browned on all sides (you may need to cook the meat in two batches to avoid crowding the pan). Transfer the meat to a large bowl.

2. Add the shallots, ginger, and garlic to pot and cook, stirring, until the shallots begin to soften, about 3 minutes.

3. Add the broth and cook, stirring and scraping up the browned bits from the bottom of the pan, for about 3 minutes.

4. Add the cooked beef back to the pan along with the water, wine, soy sauce, sugar, chili paste, cinnamon sticks, and star anise. Bring to a boil and then reduce the heat to medium low. Simmer, covered, for about 1 hour.

5. Add the carrots, turnip, and potato and continue to simmer, covered, for 45 minutes more, until the vegetables are very tender.

6. Raise the heat to medium-high and bring the pot to a boil. Stir in the cornstarch mixture and cook, stirring, for 1 minute, until the liquid thickens.

7. Add the spinach and cook, covered, until the spinach is wilted, about 3 minutes.

8. Remove and discard the cinnamon sticks and star anise.

9. Serve hot, garnished with the green onions.

Moroccan-Spiced Lamb Tagine

SERVES 4

▸ *SODIUM //* **226 MG**

MAKE AHEAD // QUICK

Tagines are traditional Moroccan stews slow cooked in specially shaped earthenware pots. This quick version boasts a heady mix of Moroccan spices, but it can be on the dinner table in just about thirty minutes.

....

2 tablespoons olive oil

1½ pounds lamb steaks (round or shoulder), cut into 1-inch pieces

½ teaspoon freshly ground pepper

4 carrots, peeled and cut into 3-inch sticks

1 medium onion, thinly sliced

3 garlic cloves, minced

1 tablespoon minced peeled fresh ginger

1 tablespoon all-purpose flour

½ cup dry white wine

2 teaspoons paprika

1 teaspoon ground cinnamon

¾ teaspoon ground coriander

½ teaspoon ground cumin

¼ teaspoon ground turmeric

¼ teaspoon cayenne pepper

¼ teaspoon ground cloves

Pinch of saffron

1 (14-ounce) can low-sodium chicken broth

1 (14-ounce) can no-salt-added diced tomatoes, drained

1 cup green beans, cut into 2-inch pieces

Juice of 1 lemon

¼ cup minced fresh flat-leaf parsley, for garnish

....

1. Heat 1 tablespoon of the oil in a Dutch oven or large stockpot over medium-high heat. Sprinkle the lamb with the pepper and add it to the pot. Cook, turning frequently, until the lamb is browned on the outside but still pink inside, about 7 minutes. Transfer the meat to a large bowl.

2. Add the remaining tablespoon of oil to the pot along with the carrots, onion, garlic, and ginger. Cook, stirring frequently, until the onion begins to soften, about 5 minutes.

3. Add the flour and cook, stirring, 1 minute more.

4. Stir in the wine and cook, scraping up any brown bits from the bottom of the pan, for about 3 minutes.

5. Add the paprika, cinnamon, coriander, cumin, turmeric, cayenne, cloves, and saffron and cook, stirring, 1 minute more.

6. Stir in the cooked lamb along with the broth, tomatoes, and green beans. Simmer until the vegetables are tender, 8 to 10 minutes.

7. Just before serving, stir in the lemon juice. Serve hot, garnished with the parsley.

CHAPTER ELEVEN

Side Dishes

S ide dishes seem to fall into two camps: simple and forgettable, or delicious and loaded with fat, salt, and calories. But it doesn't have to be that way. Whether grain- or vegetable-based, easy-to-make side dishes can deliver lots of flavor and nutrients without derailing your diet.

In this chapter, you'll find recipes for simple, delicious, and healthful sides— including grains and starchy vegetables, as well as lighter vegetable-based dishes—that will stay on your mind long after you eat them. Once you try some of these quick and easy dishes, they're likely to become regular features on your dinner table.

Lemony Snap Peas with Radishes

SERVES 4

▶ *SODIUM //* **22 MG**

LOW-FAT // QUICK

With crisp-tender snap peas, striking pink and white radishes, and the bright tang of lemon, this gorgeous side dish is as delicious as it is good for you. Both snap peas and radishes are loaded with fiber and vitamin C. Serve this bright, springy dish alongside roasted meats, especially lamb, or as part of a picnic spread.

1 pound sugar snap peas, trimmed

1 teaspoon lemon zest

2 tablespoons fresh lemon juice

1 tablespoon olive oil

1 teaspoon Dijon mustard

¾ teaspoon sugar

½ teaspoon freshly ground pepper

1 shallot, minced

4 radishes, thinly sliced

1. Fill a large bowl with ice water.

2. Bring a large pot of water to a boil. Add the snap peas and blanch until just tender, about 30 seconds. Transfer the peas from the boiling water to the ice water with a slotted spoon to stop them from cooking.

3. In a medium bowl, whisk together the lemon zest, lemon juice, oil, mustard, sugar, pepper, and shallot until well combined.

4. Drain the peas and add them to the bowl with the dressing along with the radishes. Toss to coat well. Serve immediately.

Garlicky Kale with Red Peppers

SERVES 4

▶ *SODIUM //* **60 MG**

LOW-FAT // QUICK

Kale is a true superstar of the vegetable world. It's loaded with vitamins A, C, and K (to name a few) and antioxidants, and even provides hearty doses of iron, protein, and fiber. While eating your vegetables is always a good thing, choosing kale regularly could go a long way toward keeping you strong and healthy. Here kale gets a bit of spice from jalapeño and a dash of bright color from red bell pepper. Serve it alongside a simple roast chicken or grilled meat of any kind.

2 teaspoons olive oil

2 red bell peppers, seeded and sliced

1 jalapeño, seeded and diced

1 garlic clove, minced

¼ teaspoon freshly ground pepper

1 pound kale, stems removed and leaves cut into wide ribbons

½ cup low-sodium vegetable broth

1 tablespoon fresh lemon juice

1. Heat the oil in a large, heavy skillet over medium-high heat. Add the bell peppers, jalapeño, garlic, and pepper. Cook, stirring frequently, until the peppers have softened, about 3 minutes.

2. Add the kale and broth. Reduce the heat to medium-low, cover, and cook until the kale is tender, about 10 minutes.

3. Remove the lid, increase the heat to medium, and cook until the liquid is mostly evaporated, 2 to 3 minutes.

4. Just before serving, stir in the lemon juice. Serve immediately.

Sesame-Ginger Broccoli

SERVES 4

▶ *SODIUM //* **267 MG**

LOW-FAT // QUICK

With its powerful combination of fiber and vitamins, broccoli can actually help the body reduce its level of "bad" cholesterol. This Asian-style stir-fry adds ginger, which aids in digestion, and sesame seeds, which contain lignans that lower cholesterol and blood pressure. Better still, it's delicious. Serve this side with grilled chicken or steak with Asian flavors.

½ cup low-sodium vegetable broth

1 tablespoon low-sodium soy sauce

1 tablespoon sesame oil

1 tablespoon canola oil

2 garlic cloves, minced

1 tablespoon minced peeled fresh ginger

1 pound broccoli florets, cut into bite-size pieces

1 tablespoon toasted sesame seeds

1. In a small bowl, stir together the broth, soy sauce, and sesame oil.

2. Heat the canola oil in a skillet over medium-high heat. Add the garlic and ginger and sauté for 1 minute. Add the broccoli and stir to combine.

3. Stir in the sauce mixture and bring to a boil. Reduce the heat to low, cover, and cook until the broccoli is crisp-tender, about 3 minutes. Using a slotted spoon, transfer the broccoli to a serving bowl.

4. Continue simmering the sauce until it is reduced to just a couple of tablespoons. Add the broccoli back to the pan and toss with the sauce to coat.

5. Return the broccoli to the serving bowl, sprinkle with the sesame seeds, and serve immediately.

Green Beans with Gorgonzola and Toasted Pecans

SERVES 4

▶ *SODIUM //* **205 MG**
QUICK

This savory green bean dish uses a simple steam-sauté cooking method. Just put the beans in the pan with oil and water, cover, and steam; then remove the lid, let the water evaporate, and sauté. Creamy, robust Gorgonzola cheese adds tons of flavor, and the nuts add a toasty crunch.

1 pound green beans, trimmed
¼ cup water
1 tablespoon olive oil
¼ teaspoon freshly ground pepper
⅓ cup crumbled Gorgonzola or other blue cheese
⅓ cup chopped pecans, toasted

1. Place the green beans in a large skillet along with the water and oil and bring to a boil over medium-high heat. Cover the pan, reduce the heat to medium, and simmer for about 3 minutes, until the green beans are just crisp-tender.

2. Remove the lid and continue to cook the green beans until all of the water has evaporated and the green beans begin to blister, 3 to 4 minutes more. Add the pepper and toss.

3. Place the green beans in a large serving bowl and add the Gorgonzola cheese, tossing until well combined. Sprinkle with the pecans and serve immediately.

Buttermilk Mashed Potatoes with Garlic and Chives

SERVES 4

▸ *SODIUM //* **205 MG**
LOW-FAT // QUICK

Once you taste this lightened-up version of the meat-and-potatoes standby, we're pretty sure you'll never go back to the old version. Poaching the garlic along with the potatoes infuses them with flavor. Buttermilk adds a nice tang, while still providing the creaminess you expect in mashed potatoes, and the chives add a kick of herby flavor.

2 pounds potatoes, such as Yukon Gold, peeled and cut into chunks
4 garlic cloves
2 tablespoons unsalted butter
¾ cup low-sodium chicken broth, heated
2 tablespoons nonfat buttermilk
1 tablespoon chopped chives
Freshly ground pepper

1. Place the potatoes and garlic in a large stockpot and cover with about 3 inches of water. Bring to a boil over medium-high heat. Reduce the heat to medium and cook, covered, for about 10 minutes, until the potatoes are tender. Drain the potatoes and return them to the pot.

2. Mash the potatoes and garlic using a potato masher. Add the butter.

3. Mix in ½ cup of the hot broth. If the mixture is too thick, add the remaining ¼ cup broth.

4. Add the buttermilk and chives, season with the pepper, and stir to mix well. Serve immediately.

Roasted Rosemary-Maple Sweet Potatoes

SERVES 4

▶ *SODIUM //* **22 MG**
LOW-FAT

It's impossible to overstate the healthiness of the sweet potato. In fact, along with kale, it is one of the most nutrient-dense of all the vegetables. Eat sweet potatoes on a regular basis and you'll get good doses of vitamins B_6, C, and D, plus beta-carotenes, iron, and fiber. Here sweet potatoes are roasted with olive oil and fresh rosemary, and sweetened with a dash of maple syrup. This dish makes an excellent side dish for festive holiday meals, but it's easy enough that you'll want to make it all year round.

2 pounds sweet potatoes, cut into 3 by ¼-inch sticks
2 tablespoons olive oil
½ teaspoon freshly ground pepper
2 tablespoons maple syrup
1 tablespoon minced fresh rosemary

1. Preheat the oven to 375°F.

2. On a large baking sheet, toss the sweet potatoes with the olive oil. Spread them out in a single layer and sprinkle with the pepper. Roast the sweet potatoes in the oven for 30 minutes.

3. Remove the sweet potatoes from the oven, drizzle them with the maple syrup, and sprinkle the rosemary over the top.

4. Return the sweet potatoes to the oven and roast for another 15 minutes, until the sweet potatoes are very tender. Serve immediately.

Brown Rice Pilaf with Herbs

SERVES 4

▸ *SODIUM //* **69 MG**
BUDGET-FRIENDLY // LOW-FAT

Make the switch from white rice to brown rice and you'll instantly improve the nutritional profile of your rice-based meals. Unlike white rice, brown rice still has its fiber-filled bran layer intact. This bran layer also contains healthful doses of vitamin E, magnesium, manganese, and zinc. Here we've replaced white rice with brown in a traditional rice pilaf. Lemon peel, garlic, and fresh thyme infuse the rice with flavor, and almonds add healthful fat, protein, and a welcome crunch.

1 tablespoon unsalted butter
1 shallot, chopped
1 cup long-grain brown rice
1 (2-inch) strip lemon peel
2½ cups low-sodium vegetable broth, warmed
1 garlic clove, smashed
2 sprigs fresh thyme
½ teaspoon freshly ground pepper
¼ cup slivered almonds
3 tablespoons chopped fresh flat-leaf parsley
3 green onions, thinly sliced

1. Heat the butter in a medium saucepan with a tight-fitting lid over medium heat. Add the shallot and cook, stirring frequently, until the shallot has softened, 2 to 3 minutes.

2. Add the rice and lemon peel and cook, stirring, until slightly toasted, about 2 minutes.

3. Stir in the broth, garlic, thyme, and pepper and bring to a boil.

4. Reduce the heat to low, cover, and simmer for 45 minutes or until all of the liquid has been absorbed.

5. Remove the lemon peel, thyme sprigs, and garlic clove. Stir in the almonds, parsley, and green onions. Serve immediately.

Baked Polenta with Swiss Chard

SERVES 8

▸ *SODIUM //* **398 MG**
LOW-FAT

People often forget about polenta as a whole grain, but it is one of the most enjoyable to cook with since it pairs so well with many different flavors. The smooth texture makes it a wonderful comfort food. Using the precooked variety that comes in a tube makes this dish easy to prepare.

Cooking spray
1 to 1½ cups low-sodium vegetable broth
1 (18-ounce) tube prepared polenta, diced
¾ cup (2 ounces) grated Parmesan cheese
1 egg, lightly beaten
1 tablespoon olive oil
1 small onion, diced
4 garlic cloves, minced
1 large bunch Swiss chard, stems removed and leaves cut into ribbons
2 cups water, plus more as needed
1 teaspoon red pepper flakes

1. Preheat the oven to 400°F.

2. Spray an 8 by 8-inch baking dish with cooking spray.

3. In a medium saucepan, bring 1 cup of the broth to a boil. Add the diced polenta and mash it with a wooden spoon, adding more broth as needed to achieve a smooth consistency.

4. Once the polenta is smooth and heated through, remove the pan from the heat and stir in ½ cup of the cheese and the egg.

continued ▸

5. Heat the oil a large skillet over medium-high heat. Add the onion and garlic and cook, stirring frequently, until the onion is softened, about 5 minutes.

6. Add the Swiss chard along with ½ cup of the water and cook, stirring occasionally, until the chard is wilted, about 3 minutes. Stir in the red pepper flakes.

7. Spread half of the polenta in the prepared baking dish. Next add the Swiss chard, spreading it out to cover the polenta. Spread the remaining polenta over the top and sprinkle with the remaining ¼ cup cheese.

8. Bake the polenta in the oven for about 20 minutes, until bubbling.

9. Remove from the oven and let sit for 10 minutes before serving.

Whole-Wheat Couscous with Carrots and Raisins

SERVES 8

▸ *SODIUM* // **76 MG**
LOW-FAT // *QUICK*

Whole-wheat couscous is made from durum flour, which is high in protein. It is also low in fat, high in fiber, and provides carbohydrates for energy. It's a good addition to any healthful diet. The carrots add vibrant color and a lot of beta-carotene while the raisins provide more energy and antioxidants.

4 cups low-sodium vegetable broth

2 medium carrots, diced small

2½ cups whole-wheat couscous

1½ cups raisins

1 cup slivered almonds, toasted

4 green onions, chopped

2 tablespoons unsalted butter, at room temperature

1. In a large saucepan, bring the broth to a boil. Reduce the heat to medium, add the carrots, and simmer until the carrots are tender, about 5 minutes.

2. Remove the saucepan from the heat and stir in the couscous and raisins. Cover and let stand for 15 minutes, until the couscous is tender and the liquid has been absorbed.

3. Stir in the almonds, green onions, and butter. Serve immediately.

Quinoa with Caramelized Onions and Mushrooms

SERVES 4

▸ *SODIUM //* **249 MG**
BUDGET-FRIENDLY // LOW-FAT

Quinoa is trendy among health-conscious types for a reason. It is rich in protein and a great source of fiber and magnesium, which helps to lower blood pressure and keep blood sugar stable.

1¼ cups low-sodium chicken or vegetable broth
1 cup quinoa, rinsed
1 tablespoon olive oil
2 medium yellow onions, thinly sliced
½ pound cremini or button mushrooms, sliced
¼ teaspoon freshly ground pepper
¼ cup minced fresh flat-leaf parsley, for garnish

1. In a medium saucepan, bring the broth to a boil over medium-high heat. Reduce the heat to low and add the quinoa. Cook, covered, for about 15 minutes, until the quinoa is tender and the liquid has been absorbed. Remove it from the heat.

2. Heat the oil in a large, heavy skillet over medium heat. Add the onions and cook, stirring frequently, until the onions are very soft and caramelized, about 30 minutes. Reduce the heat to medium-low if the onions seem to be cooking too quickly. You can also add a bit of water to keep the onions from burning or sticking to the pan.

3. Add the mushrooms and pepper and raise the heat to medium-high. Cook, stirring, until the mushrooms are tender, about 5 minutes more.

4. Stir the cooked quinoa into the onion mixture and cook, stirring, just until heated through. Serve immediately, garnished with the parsley.

CHAPTER TWELVE

Fish and Seafood Entrées

I f you are concerned about your risk of heart disease, fish and seafood should make frequent appearances on your menu. In fact, adding one to two servings of fish a week could significantly reduce your risk of dying of a heart attack, thanks to the high levels of omega-3 fatty acids that make fish so healthful.

Because fish and seafood tend to have delicate flavors of their own, it doesn't take much to spice them up and turn them into delectable meals. This chapter includes recipes for both fish and shellfish, which are low in fat and sodium but full of delicious flavor.

Grilled Halibut with Mango Salsa

SERVES 4

▶ *SODIUM* // **123 MG**
LOW-FAT // QUICK

Halibut is a meaty and flavorful fish that is loaded with protein and magnesium, vitamins B_6 and B_{12}, and omega-3 fatty acids. It's also well suited to grilling, which is a great healthful cooking method. This recipe is full of tropical flavors, and it is perfect for a barbecue on a warm summer evening. A fish grilling basket is a wise investment. This inexpensive gadget will keep your fish from falling through the slats of the grill and make it easy to flip.

For the salsa:
2 medium mangos, pitted, peeled, and diced
1 medium red bell pepper, seeded and diced
2 green onions, thinly sliced
2 jalapeños, seeded and diced
1 garlic clove, minced
Juice of 2 limes
1 tablespoon chopped fresh oregano

For the fish:
Cooking spray
1 tablespoon fresh lemon juice
1 tablespoon olive oil
½ teaspoon paprika
1 garlic clove, minced
4 (6-ounce) skinless halibut fillets
½ teaspoon freshly ground pepper

To make the salsa:

1. In a medium mixing bowl, combine all the ingredients. Stir well.

To make the fish:

1. Preheat a barbecue or gas grill to medium-high heat.

2. Spray a fish grilling basket with cooking spray.

3. In a small bowl, stir together the lemon juice, oil, paprika, and garlic. Place the fish in a baking dish and pour the sauce over it. Turn the fish to coat it on all sides. Cover and let the fish marinate for about 15 minutes.

4. Take the fish out of the marinade and discard the marinade. Sprinkle the fish with the pepper, and grill in the fish grilling basket on the barbecue or grill for about 3 minutes per side, until it is cooked through and flakes easily.

5. Serve the fish topped with the mango salsa.

Seared Salmon with Cilantro-Lime Pesto

SERVES 4

▶ *SODIUM //* **205 MG**
QUICK

It's common knowledge that salmon is one of the healthiest proteins around, providing more than half of the recommended daily allowance of omega-3 fatty acids in just one 6-ounce serving. It's also one of the most delicious and easy-to-prepare fishes, due to its meaty flesh and relatively high fat content. Here the pretty pink fish is paired with a bright green sauce that's loaded with the flavors of cilantro, lime, and Parmesan cheese. Serve it alongside sautéed snap peas (try the Lemony Snap Peas with Radishes on page 135) for a beautiful spring meal.

....

For the pesto:
2 garlic cloves
1 cup fresh cilantro leaves
⅓ cup (1½ ounces) grated Parmesan cheese
1 teaspoon lime zest
2 tablespoons fresh lime juice
2 tablespoons olive oil

For the fish:
Cooking spray
4 (6-ounce) salmon fillets, with skin
¼ teaspoon freshly ground pepper

....

To make the pesto:

1. Place the garlic in a food processor and pulse to mince. Add the cilantro, cheese, lime zest, and lime juice and pulse until finely chopped.

2. With the processor running, drizzle in the oil until well combined.

To make the fish:

1. Coat a nonstick skillet with cooking spray and heat it over medium-high heat. Sprinkle the salmon with pepper and place it in the pan skin side down. Cook the salmon until the skin begins to brown, 5 to 6 minutes.

2. Turn the fish over and cook the other side until the fish is cooked through and flakes easily with a fork, about 6 minutes more.

3. Serve immediately with a dollop of the pesto on top.

Pecan-Crusted Honey-Dijon Salmon

SERVES 6

▶ *SODIUM //* **224 MG**
QUICK

With its crunchy, nutty coating and sweet-spicy honey mustard sauce, this easy-to-make dish is sure to become a favorite. It takes less than twenty minutes to prepare, making it a perfect choice for a busy workday evening. Serve it with quick sautéed green beans or steamed broccoli and quinoa for an easy meal that hits all the right notes.

Cooking spray
3 tablespoons Dijon mustard
1 tablespoon olive oil
1 tablespoon honey
½ cup finely chopped pecans
½ cup fresh bread crumbs
6 (4-ounce) salmon fillets
1 tablespoon minced fresh parsley, for garnish

1. Preheat the oven to 400°F.

2. Spray a large baking dish lightly with cooking spray.

3. In a small bowl, combine the mustard, oil, and honey.

4. In a separate small bowl, combine the pecans and bread crumbs.

5. Arrange the fillets on a large baking sheet. Brush the fillets first with the honey-mustard mixture, and then top them with the pecan mixture, dividing it equally.

6. Bake the salmon in the oven until it is cooked through and flakes easily with a fork, about 15 minutes.

7. Serve immediately, garnished with the parsley.

Seared Trout with Cherry Tomatoes and Bacon

SERVES 4

▶ *SODIUM //* **338 MG**
QUICK

Bacon and trout is a classic flavor combination, and for good reason. It's delicious, but it's usually very high in sodium. Here we've used just two slices of bacon. You still get the delicious smokiness, but with very little sodium per serving. Switch to turkey bacon for even lower sodium. Sweet-tart cherry tomatoes and fresh herbs keep the dish tasting fresh and light.

2 slices bacon
1 pint cherry tomatoes, halved
1 garlic clove, minced
1 teaspoon freshly ground pepper
1 tablespoon minced fresh thyme
Cooking spray
4 (6-ounce) trout fillets
4 lemon wedges, for garnish

1. Heat a medium skillet over medium-high heat. Add the bacon and cook, turning once, until crisp, 5 to 7 minutes. Transfer the bacon to a paper towel-lined plate to drain, and then crumble it. Drain off all but about 1 tablespoon of bacon fat from the pan.

2. Add the tomatoes, garlic, and ½ teaspoon of the pepper to the pan and cook, stirring, until the tomatoes just begin to break down, about 3 minutes. Remove the pan from the heat, and stir in the crumbled bacon and the thyme.

continued ▶

3. Spray a large nonstick skillet with cooking spray and heat it over medium-high heat. Sprinkle the remaining ½ teaspoon of pepper over the fish and add them to the pan (you may need to cook the fish in two batches to avoid overcrowding the pan). Cook the fish, turning once, until it is cooked through and flakes easily with a fork, 2 to 3 minutes per side.

4. Transfer the fish fillets to serving plates and serve topped with the tomato mixture and lemon wedges on the side.

Fish Tacos with Chipotle Cream

SERVES 4

▶ *SODIUM //* **255 MG**
QUICK

Tacos are often loaded with fatty meats, cheese, and other no-nos for those on restricted diets. Here we use baked red snapper, which is one of the lighter fishes, topped with crunchy cabbage and a low-fat but flavorful cream sauce. Serve these quick, healthful tacos with a crisp salad of lettuce, sliced radishes, diced avocado, and tomatoes with a lime vinaigrette and bottles of cold Mexican beer.

....

For the chipotle cream:

3 tablespoons reduced-fat mayonnaise

3 tablespoons reduced-fat sour cream

1 teaspoon ground chipotle

1 teaspoon lime zest

1½ teaspoons fresh lime juice

¼ cup chopped fresh cilantro

For the tacos:

1 teaspoon ground cumin

1 teaspoon ground coriander

1 teaspoon mild chili powder

½ teaspoon smoked paprika

⅛ teaspoon garlic powder

1½ pounds red snapper fillets, cut into 2-inch strips

Cooking spray

8 (6-inch) corn tortillas

2 cups shredded cabbage

....

To make the chipotle cream:

1. Combine all the ingredients and stir well.

continued ▶

To make the tacos:

1. Preheat the oven to 425°F.

2. In a small bowl, combine the cumin, coriander, chili powder, paprika, and garlic powder. Dust the fish all over with the spice mixture.

3. Spray a large baking sheet lightly with cooking spray. Arrange the fish in a single layer on the baking sheet and bake in the oven until the fish is cooked through and flakes easily with a fork, 8 to 10 minutes.

4. Wrap the tortillas in aluminum foil and heat them in the oven for a few minutes to warm them.

5. Remove the tortillas from the oven and place 2 on each of 4 dinner plates. Top each tortilla with the fish and the cabbage, dividing it equally. Drizzle each taco with a bit of the chipotle cream and serve immediately.

Spicy Grilled Prawn Skewers with Cucumber-Cashew Salad

SERVES 4

▸ *SODIUM* // **97 MG**
QUICK

Healthful, low-calorie, quick-cooking prawns are well suited to grilling. Here they get a spicy rub and are served atop a refreshing cucumber salad to cool the fire. This is a perfect meal for a backyard barbecue.

....

For the cucumber salad:
2 medium cucumbers, peeled, seeded, and diced
½ cup coarsely chopped unsalted roasted cashews
2 green onions, thinly sliced
2 tablespoons olive oil
1 tablespoon fresh lemon juice
¼ cup chopped fresh flat-leaf parsley

For the prawns:
1 large serrano chili, seeded and finely minced
1 tablespoon olive oil
1 teaspoon ground cumin
1 teaspoon ground chili powder
1 to 1½ pounds prawns, peeled and deveined

....

To make the cucumber salad:

1. In a large bowl, toss together the cucumbers, cashews, green onions, oil, lemon juice, and parsley.

To make the prawns:

1. Preheat the grill to medium-high.

continued ▸

2. Soak 4 wooden skewers in water.

3. In a large bowl, combine the serrano chili, oil, cumin, and chili powder. Add the prawns to the bowl and toss to coat.

4. Thread the prawns onto the skewers.

5. Grill the prawns for about 3 minutes per side, until they are pink and cooked through.

6. To serve, divide the cucumber salad among 4 serving plates. Top each with 1 skewer and serve immediately.

Spaghetti with Broiled Shrimp Scampi

SERVES 4

▶ *SODIUM //* **482 MG**
QUICK

Surprisingly easy but as delicious as any Italian restaurant's shrimp scampi, this dish pairs plump shrimp with lots of lemon. It can be made in about twenty minutes, making it a great weeknight dish, but it's also impressive enough to serve to company. Add a crisp green salad with a tangy vinaigrette and a bottle of dry white wine, and your party has just begun.

12 ounces dried spaghetti
1 tablespoon olive oil
3 tablespoons chopped fresh parsley
1½ pounds jumbo shrimp, peeled and deveined
2 tablespoons unsalted butter, melted
2 garlic cloves, minced
¼ teaspoon freshly ground pepper
2 tablespoons fresh lemon juice

1. Preheat the broiler.

2. Cook the spaghetti according to the package directions (omitting the salt). Drain.

3. Toss the spaghetti with the oil and 2 tablespoons of the parsley, cover, and keep warm.

4. In a large baking dish, toss the shrimp with the butter, garlic, and pepper. Broil under the broiler, turning once, until the shrimp are pink and cooked through, 2 to 3 minutes per side. Remove the shrimp from the broiler and toss them with the lemon juice.

5. Divide the spaghetti evenly among 4 shallow serving bowls. Top with the shrimp, dividing it equally. Spoon a bit of the sauce from the baking dish over each portion and serve immediately, garnished with the remaining 1 tablespoon of parsley.

Seared Sea Scallops with Paprika Brown Butter

SERVES 4

▶ *SODIUM //* **416 MG**
QUICK

Scallops are a good source of vitamin B_{12}, omega-3 fatty acids, and magnesium, all of which promote cardiovascular health. With a mild flavor and succulent texture, scallops are loved even by people who aren't usually crazy about shellfish. Serve these elegant scallops alongside roasted asparagus and wild rice pilaf for a celebratory meal or dinner party.

3 tablespoons unsalted butter

1½ pounds jumbo sea scallops

¼ teaspoon freshly ground pepper

1 teaspoon minced fresh garlic

3 tablespoons fresh lemon juice

2 (5-ounce) packages baby spinach

¼ teaspoon paprika

⅛ teaspoon cayenne pepper

2 tablespoons low-sodium chicken broth

¼ cup pine nuts, toasted

1. In a large skillet over medium-high heat, melt 2 tablespoons of the butter.

2. Pat the scallops dry with a paper towel, season them with the pepper, and then add them to the pan. Cook until nicely golden brown on the bottom, about 2 minutes, and then flip them over and cook until golden brown on the second side, about 2 minutes more. Transfer the scallops to a plate and keep warm.

3. Melt the remaining 1 tablespoon of butter in the skillet and add the garlic and spinach. Cook for about 2 minutes, until just wilted. Remove the spinach and garlic from the pan and keep warm.

4. Add the lemon juice, paprika, and cayenne to the pan and simmer for about 15 seconds.

5. Add the broth. Simmer, scraping up any bits from the pan, for about 3 minutes, until the sauce is reduced.

6. Return the scallops, along with any juices, to the skillet and cook over low heat until heated through.

7. Arrange the spinach on 4 serving plates, dividing it equally. Top each with scallops, dividing them equally. Drizzle the sauce over the scallops and sprinkle the pine nuts on top. Serve immediately.

Classic Crab Cakes with Red Pepper Aioli

SERVES 4

▶ *SODIUM //* **346 MG**
LOW-FAT

Crab cakes are often either laden with gloppy mayonnaise and loaded with salt or so full of herbs and vegetables that you can barely taste the crab. This recipe solves both problems. Big pieces of succulent crabmeat are held together by just a touch of reduced-fat mayonnaise and seasoned with a dash of spices, a squeeze of lime, and a sprinkling of fresh herbs. These are quick and easy to make, low in fat and sodium, and full of crabmeat and flavorful herbs and spices. They are a simple and delicious everyday meal or an elegant dish for a special occasion.

....

For the crab cakes:
½ cup panko bread crumbs
1 egg
1 egg white, beaten
2 green onions, thinly sliced
2 tablespoons finely chopped red bell pepper
2 tablespoons minced fresh parsley
1 tablespoon reduced-fat mayonnaise
Juice of ½ lime
1 teaspoon Old Bay Seasoning
½ teaspoon freshly ground pepper
9 ounces lump crabmeat
Cooking spray

For the aioli:
¼ cup nonfat plain Greek yogurt
2 tablespoons reduced-fat mayonnaise
¼ cup jarred roasted red bell pepper (packed in water),
    drained, seeded, and chopped

....

To make the crab cakes:

1. In a large mixing bowl, combine the bread crumbs, egg, egg white, green onions, bell pepper, parsley, mayonnaise, lime juice, Old Bay Seasoning, and pepper and stir to mix well.

2. Using your hands, gently fold in the crabmeat, being careful not to break up the large pieces.

3. Shape into 8 equal-size patties and refrigerate for 30 to 60 minutes.

4. Preheat the oven to 400°F.

5. Spray a large baking sheet with cooking spray.

6. Arrange the chilled crab cakes on the baking sheet and spray lightly with cooking spray. Bake for about 10 minutes on each side.

To make the aioli:

1. In a small bowl, combine the yogurt, mayonnaise, and roasted pepper. Stir to mix well.

2. Serve the crab cakes hot, garnished with a dollop of the aioli.

Mixed Seafood Grill with Romesco Sauce

SERVES 4

▶ *SODIUM //* **402 MG**
QUICK

This stunning dish is a healthful alternative to the usual barbecue fare. A fish-grilling basket makes it a cinch to create. If you don't have one, you can put the seafood and fish on soaked wooden skewers to keep them from falling through the slats on your barbecue and make them easier to flip.

For the sauce:
1 (7-ounce) jar roasted red peppers (packed in water), drained
2 large tomatoes, quartered
¼ cup unsalted almonds, toasted
2 garlic cloves
2 tablespoons minced fresh parsley
1 tablespoon sherry vinegar
1 teaspoon paprika
½ teaspoon freshly ground pepper
2 tablespoons olive oil

For the seafood:
Cooking spray
½ pound shrimp, peeled and deveined
½ pound sea scallops
½ pound whole squid, separated into bodies and tentacles
1 (10-ounce) firm fish fillet, such as haddock or snapper, cut into strips
2 tablespoons olive oil
1 teaspoon dried oregano
½ teaspoon freshly ground pepper
2 tablespoons minced fresh flat-leaf parsley, for garnish
2 lemons, cut into wedges, for garnish

To make the sauce:

1. Combine the red peppers, tomatoes, almonds, garlic, parsley, vinegar, paprika, and pepper in a food processor and process to a fairly smooth paste.

2. With the processor running, drizzle in the oil and process until well combined. If the mixture is too thick, add water, 1 tablespoon at a time, to achieve the desired consistency.

To make the seafood:

1. Preheat a grill or barbecue to medium-high heat.

2. Spray a seafood grilling basket, if using, lightly with cooking spray. Soak 12 bamboo skewers in water if you don't have a grilling basket.

3. In a large bowl, toss the shrimp, scallops, squid, and fish with the oil, oregano, and pepper. Skewer the seafood, if necessary.

4. Place the seafood on the grill (either skewered or in the grilling basket) and cook, turning as needed, until all of the pieces are charred and cooked through. Squid will take about 2 minutes per side, shrimp about 3 minutes per side, and fish about 4 minutes per side, so you may want to grill in batches.

5. Serve the seafood immediately on a large platter, garnished with the parsley and the lemon wedges. Offer one large bowl of the Romesco sauce for dipping, or give each diner an individual dipping bowl of sauce.

CHAPTER THIRTEEN

Poultry, Pork, and Beef Entrées

For many, meat entrées are the central focus of their diets, for good or bad. Too often, meat dishes are heavy on fat, calories, and sodium. But it doesn't have to be this way. Chicken and turkey, cooked without the skin, are very low in fat. Certain cuts of pork, too, are naturally low in fat. And even beef, if you choose the right cut and use it sparingly, can be part of a healthful diet.

In this chapter, you'll find recipes for seared, braised, grilled, and roasted meat entrées—chicken, turkey, pork, and beef—that will keep you both satisfied and on track.

Pan-Roasted Chicken Breast in Dijon Sauce

SERVES 4

▸ *SODIUM //* **459 MG**

BUDGET-FRIENDLY // MAKE AHEAD

Roast chicken is a welcome comfort food during the colder months. This simple version gets a lot of flavor from Dijon mustard and fresh herbs. It's wonderful served with a salad and roasted or mashed potatoes. It is an equally delicious leftover used for salads or sandwiches. Save the carcass, too, and use it to make a rich homemade chicken stock.

....

1 (4-pound) whole chicken

2 lemons, cut in half

6 large garlic cloves

1 tablespoon unsalted butter, at room temperature

4 tablespoons Dijon mustard

1 tablespoon minced fresh thyme

½ teaspoon freshly ground pepper

¾ cup low-sodium chicken broth

½ cup dry white wine

3 tablespoons reduced-fat sour cream

1 tablespoon finely chopped fresh chives

....

1. Preheat the oven to 450°F.

2. Place the chicken in a large oven-safe skillet, such as a cast iron skillet. Place the lemons and garlic inside the cavity of the chicken. Rub the butter underneath the skin of the breasts. Coat the outside of the chicken with 2 tablespoons of the mustard. Sprinkle the chicken with the thyme and pepper.

3. Roast the chicken in the oven for 50 to 60 minutes, until it reaches an internal temperature of 165°F on an instant-read thermometer.

4. Remove the chicken from the oven and transfer it to a platter or cutting board. Carefully remove 3 of the garlic cloves. Tent the chicken loosely with foil and let it rest while you prepare the sauce.

5. Place the skillet on the stove over medium-high heat. Smash the garlic cloves with the side of a knife and add them to the drippings in the skillet. Add the broth and wine and cook, stirring and scraping up any brown bits, for 3 minutes.

6. Stir in the sour cream and boil for about 1 minute, until slightly thickened. Stir in the remaining 2 tablespoons of mustard and the chives.

7. Carve the chicken and serve it with the sauce.

Braised Chicken with Tomato Sauce and Olives

SERVES 6

▶ *SODIUM //* **360 MG**
QUICK

This simple dish—chicken thighs braised in a rich tomato sauce fortified with olives, capers, fresh herbs, and plenty of garlic—is Italian-style comfort food at its best. While people on restricted diets often choose chicken breast, the thigh meat actually contains more iron and other nutrients. By braising it without the skin, you get rich, moist meat without too much fat.

....

2 tablespoons olive oil
6 skinless chicken thighs
½ teaspoon freshly ground pepper
1 medium onion, diced
3 garlic cloves, minced
¼ cup dry white wine
2 cups low-sodium chicken broth
2 tablespoons capers, drained
¼ cup sliced pitted cured green olives
1 tablespoon chopped fresh oregano
1 (28-ounce) can no-salt-added diced tomatoes, with juice
2 tablespoons chopped fresh flat-leaf parsley, for garnish

....

1. Heat the oil in a large skillet over medium-high heat. Sprinkle the chicken with pepper, add it to the skillet, and cook, turning once, until browned on both sides, about 4 minutes total (cook the chicken in batches if necessary to avoid overcrowding the pan). Transfer the chicken to a plate.

2. Reduce the heat to medium. Add the onion and garlic to the pan and cook, stirring frequently, until the onion is softened, about 4 minutes.

3. Stir in the wine and simmer, stirring and scraping up any browned bits from the bottom of the pan, for about 3 minutes, until the liquid is reduced by about half. Add the broth, capers, olives, oregano, and tomatoes with their juice.

4. Reduce the heat to medium-low, return the chicken thighs to the pan, and cover them with the sauce. Simmer, uncovered, for about 20 minutes, until the chicken is fully cooked.

5. Serve the chicken with the sauce spooned over, garnished with the parsley.

Chinese Chicken and Veggie Stir-Fry

SERVES 6

▶ *SODIUM //* **574 MG**
LOW-FAT // QUICK

Stir-fries are a great way to get lots of vegetables into your meal. Here we combine disease-fighting broccoli, carrots, onions, cabbage, and snow peas with lean, protein-rich chicken breast. For a variation, try your own combinations. You might spice it up with a dash of chili paste or add fresh herbs like cilantro or basil, or top it with toasted cashews or peanuts for added crunch.

3 tablespoons Chinese cooking wine, rice wine (mirin), or dry sherry

4 tablespoons low-sodium soy sauce

1 tablespoon cornstarch

1 pound skinless, boneless chicken breast, cut into bite-size pieces

5 tablespoons water

2 tablespoons honey

2 tablespoons unseasoned rice vinegar

2 garlic cloves, minced

1 tablespoon peeled minced fresh ginger

1 tablespoon vegetable oil

2 cups broccoli florets, finely chopped

1 medium onion, diced

2 medium carrots, peeled and diced

5 cups green cabbage, shredded

2 cups snow peas, trimmed and halved crosswise

3 green onions, thinly sliced, for garnish

1. In a medium bowl, whisk together the wine, 2 tablespoons of the soy sauce, and the cornstarch to make the marinade. Add the chicken and stir to coat. Let stand for 15 minutes.

2. In a small bowl, combine the remaining 2 tablespoons of soy sauce, 3 tablespoons of the water, the honey, vinegar, garlic, and ginger.

3. Heat the oil in a large nonstick skillet or wok over medium-high heat. Add the broccoli, onion, carrots, and remaining 2 tablespoons of water. Cook until the broccoli is crisp-tender, about 5 minutes.

4. Add the cabbage and sauté for 2 minutes more, until the cabbage is wilted. Add the snow peas and cook for 2 more minutes. Transfer the vegetables to a large bowl.

5. Add the chicken to the skillet along with the marinade and cook, stirring occasionally, until cooked through, about 3 minutes.

6. Add the sauce mixture and return the vegetables to the pan. Stir to mix well and cook until everything is heated through and the sauce has thickened, about 3 minutes more.

7. Serve hot, garnished with the green onions.

Oven-Fried Buttermilk Chicken

SERVES 6

▶ *SODIUM //* **329 MG**

LOW-FAT // MAKE AHEAD

Who says you have to give up fried chicken in order to eat healthfully? This oven-baked version will fill that craving with gusto. Marinating the chicken in low-fat buttermilk makes it super-tender (the longer you marinate it, the more tender it will be). The buttermilk also helps the spices in the marinade permeate the meat so that it's extra flavorful. Cornflakes provide a crispy crunch without deep-frying.

⅔ cup low-fat buttermilk

1 teaspoon paprika

½ teaspoon cayenne pepper

½ teaspoon garlic powder

½ teaspoon onion powder

½ teaspoon freshly ground pepper

1 (3½-pound) whole chicken, cut into 8 pieces (breast, thigh, leg, and wing)

½ cup all-purpose flour

4 cups cornflakes, crushed

1. In a large bowl, combine the buttermilk, paprika, cayenne, garlic powder, onion powder, and pepper. Add the chicken and turn to coat. Cover and refrigerate the chicken for at least 1 hour, preferably overnight.

2. Preheat the oven to 425°F.

3. Place a wire rack on a large baking sheet.

4. Put the flour and the crushed cornflakes in separate shallow bowls.

5. Remove the chicken from the buttermilk mixture, letting the excess drain back into the bowl. Dredge the chicken in the flour. Dunk the floured chicken back into the buttermilk mixture and then into the cornflakes, rolling to coat the chicken completely.

6. Place the chicken on the wire rack and bake in the oven until nicely browned and cooked through, about 30 minutes. Serve hot.

Greek Turkey Burgers with Feta Cheese

SERVES 4

▸ *SODIUM* // **359 MG**
QUICK

This healthful take on the hamburger gives you all the flavors of a Greek salad and all the fun of a burger in one dish.

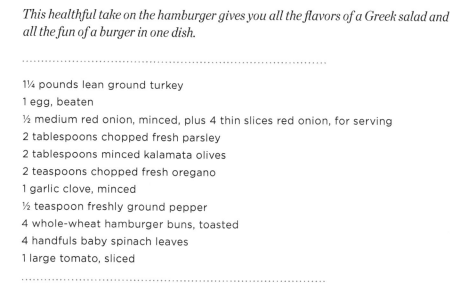

1¼ pounds lean ground turkey
1 egg, beaten
½ medium red onion, minced, plus 4 thin slices red onion, for serving
2 tablespoons chopped fresh parsley
2 tablespoons minced kalamata olives
2 teaspoons chopped fresh oregano
1 garlic clove, minced
½ teaspoon freshly ground pepper
4 whole-wheat hamburger buns, toasted
4 handfuls baby spinach leaves
1 large tomato, sliced

1. In a large mixing bowl, combine the turkey, egg, minced onion, parsley, olives, oregano, garlic, and pepper and mix well. Shape the mixture into 4 equal-size patties, about ½ inch thick.

2. Heat a barbecue or grill to medium-high heat, or heat a nonstick skillet over medium-high heat. Cook the burgers for about 4 minutes per side, until cooked through and browned on the outside.

3. Serve the burgers inside the bun with spinach, tomato, and a slice of red onion. Offer condiments such as mayonnaise, ketchup, or mustard, as desired.

Savory Turkey Meatloaf with Mushrooms

SERVES 4

▸ *SODIUM //* **390 MG**

MAKE AHEAD

Once you try this moist, flavorful, and light meatloaf, we suspect you'll never go back to the heavier beef version. Serve it alongside pureed cauliflower or mashed potatoes and sautéed green beans, or chill it and tuck thick slices between toasted whole-wheat bread with additional ketchup and crisp lettuce leaves.

Cooking spray
1 tablespoon canola oil
1 medium onion, minced
2 garlic cloves, minced
½ pound cremini or button mushrooms, minced
½ teaspoon freshly ground pepper
1¼ pounds lean ground turkey
1 cup panko bread crumbs
2 eggs, lightly beaten
½ cup low-sodium ketchup
1 tablespoon Worcestershire sauce

1. Preheat the oven to 400°F.

2. Line a baking sheet with aluminum foil sprayed with cooking spray.

3. Heat the oil in a large skillet over medium-high heat. Add the onion and garlic and cook, stirring, until the onion begins to soften, about 3 minutes.

4. Reduce the heat to medium, add the mushrooms and pepper, and cook, stirring frequently, until the mushrooms and onion are soft and most of the liquid has evaporated, about 8 minutes. Set aside to cool.

5. In a large mixing bowl, combine the turkey, bread crumbs, eggs, ¼ cup of the ketchup, and the Worcestershire sauce. When the mushroom mixture is cool enough, add it to the turkey mixture and mix well.

6. Transfer the mixture to the prepared baking sheet and form it into a loaf shape, about 8 inches long and 4 inches wide. Spread the remaining ¼ cup of ketchup over the top.

7. Bake the meatloaf in the oven for 45 to 50 minutes, until it is cooked through. Let it stand 5 minutes before slicing.

8. Serve the meatloaf hot or refrigerate it and use it for sandwiches.

Pan-Seared Turkey Cutlets with Rosemary-Orange Glaze

SERVES 4

▶ *SODIUM* // **203 MG**

BUDGET-FRIENDLY // LOW-FAT // QUICK

We mostly think of turkey as being either a whole turkey cooked on special holidays like Thanksgiving, or sliced as deli meat. But turkey breast cutlets are a great choice for weeknight dinners. They are quick cooking, very low in fat, and pair well with whatever flavors you crave.

¼ cup fresh orange juice

2 tablespoons balsamic vinegar

1 tablespoon low-sodium soy sauce

1 tablespoon honey

2 teaspoons minced fresh rosemary

1 garlic clove, minced

½ teaspoon freshly ground pepper

1 pound skinless turkey breast cutlets, cut about ½ inch thick

Cooking spray

1. In a medium bowl, combine the orange juice, vinegar, soy sauce, honey, rosemary, garlic, and pepper and mix well.

2. Add the cutlets to the bowl and turn to coat. Let stand for 15 minutes.

3. Spray a nonstick skillet with cooking spray and heat it over medium heat. Remove the cutlets from the marinade, reserving the marinade, and cook, turning once, until browned on both sides and cooked through, 8 to 10 minutes. Transfer the cutlets to a plate and keep warm.

4. Add the reserved marinade to the skillet and bring it to a boil. Simmer, stirring frequently, until the sauce is reduced to a thick glaze, 5 to 7 minutes.

5. Serve the cutlets drizzled with the sauce.

Roast Pork Tenderloin with Fig Glaze

SERVES 4

▶ *SODIUM //* **506 MG**
LOW-FAT

Bite for bite, pork tenderloin has less fat than chicken breast, making it a great source of lean protein. A serving of this flavorful meat also provides a good dose of selenium and zinc. Herbes de Provence is a blend of herbs that most often includes savory, fennel, basil, thyme, and lavender. Here this mix adds floral notes to a sweet and rich fig glaze that is used to flavor the lean pork tenderloin.

1 (1-pound) pork tenderloin
1 tablespoon herbes de Provence
½ teaspoon freshly ground pepper
⅓ cup fig jam
⅓ cup honey
2 tablespoons low-sodium soy sauce
1 tablespoon rice vinegar

1. Season the tenderloin with the herbes de Provence and pepper.

2. Combine the jam, honey, soy sauce, and vinegar in a small saucepan over medium heat. Bring it to a simmer, and then remove it from the heat.

3. Transfer half of the glaze to a small bowl and set aside. Use the remaining glaze to marinate the meat, either in a bowl or a large, sealable plastic bag in the refrigerator for 1 hour.

4. Preheat the oven to 425°F.

continued ▶

5. Remove the tenderloin from the marinade, discard the marinade, and place the tenderloin on a roasting rack or in a roasting pan. Cook in the oven for about 15 minutes, or until it reaches an internal temperature of 145°F on an instant-read thermometer.

6. Transfer the meat to a cutting board, tent loosely with foil, and let it stand for 10 minutes.

7. Meanwhile, bring the remaining glaze to a simmer in small saucepan over medium-high heat. Reduce the heat to medium-low and simmer until the glaze thickens, 5 to 10 minutes.

8. Slice the tenderloin into ¼-inch-thick pieces and serve with the glaze spooned over the top.

Pork Chops with Green Peppercorn Sauce

SERVES 4

▶ *SODIUM //* **290 MG**
QUICK

Green peppercorns are simply black peppercorns that are harvested before they are ripe. They are usually sold in jars of vinegary brine and they have an unusual sharp and tangy flavor. You can find green peppercorns in most supermarkets (look for them near the capers and olives), but you can substitute a teaspoon of cracked black peppercorns in this dish, if you prefer.

4 (4-ounce) boneless pork chops, ½ inch thick, trimmed
½ teaspoon freshly ground pepper
3 tablespoons all-purpose flour
2 tablespoons extra-virgin olive oil
1 medium shallot, minced
1 garlic clove, smashed
½ cup brandy
¼ cup reduced-fat sour cream
2 tablespoons low-sodium chicken broth
2 tablespoons green peppercorns in brine, drained

1. Dust the pork chops on both sides with the pepper and then dredge them in the flour.

2. Heat the oil in a large skillet over medium-high heat. Add the pork chops and cook, turning once, until they are browned and cooked through, about 3 minutes on each side (you may have to cook the chops in 2 batches to avoid crowding the pan). Place the cooked chops on a plate and tent loosely with aluminum foil.

continued ▶

3. Reduce the heat to medium-low, add the shallot and the garlic to the pan, and cook, stirring frequently, until the shallot is softened, about 3 minutes.

4. Add the brandy to the pan and cook, stirring frequently, for 2 minutes, until most of the brandy evaporates.

5. Stir in the sour cream, broth, and peppercorns. Simmer, stirring, until the sauce thickens and is well combined.

6. Serve the pork chops immediately, with the sauce spooned over the top.

Chinese Pork Stir-Fry

SERVES 4

▶ *SODIUM //* **437 MG**
LOW-FAT // QUICK

Stir-fries are always a favorite on busy weeknights. They're quick to prepare, full of flavor, and you can cover protein and vegetables in one pot. This low-fat stir-fry takes only minutes to prepare, but it is long on flavor. Serve it over steamed brown rice or noodles, if desired.

2 teaspoons canola oil
1 teaspoon Asian sesame oil
1 (1-pound) pork tenderloin, cut into 1 by 2–inch strips
2 garlic cloves, minced
1 teaspoon minced peeled fresh ginger
1 teaspoon chili paste
1 red bell pepper, seeded and cut into strips
¼ cup low-sodium chicken broth
1½ tablespoons low-sodium soy sauce
1 tablespoon all-natural no-salt-added peanut butter
4 green onions, thinly sliced

1. Heat the oils in a large nonstick skillet over medium-high heat. Add the pork, garlic, ginger, and chili paste and cook, stirring frequently, for about 2 minutes.

2. Add the bell pepper and cook, stirring, until the pepper begins to soften, about 2 minutes more.

3. Stir in the broth, soy sauce, and peanut butter and bring to a boil. Reduce the heat to low and cook, stirring, just until the sauce begins to thicken, about 1 minute more.

4. Stir in the green onions and serve immediately.

Pan-Seared Pork Medallions with Apples, Shallots, and Sage

SERVES 4

▸ *SODIUM //* **127 MG**

QUICK

With its classic flavor combination, this comfort dish is sure to satisfy. Pork medallions are cut from the lean tenderloin, which keeps this dish from being overly fatty. Be sure to choose an apple that is good for cooking, such as Gravenstein, Rome, or Golden Delicious. Serve with braised cabbage and a bit of bacon to complete the classic flavor combination.

2 tablespoons olive oil

4 (6-ounce) boneless center-cut pork medallions

½ teaspoon freshly ground pepper

2 medium shallots, sliced

2 tablespoons apple cider vinegar

1 tablespoon unsalted butter

1 medium apple, peeled, halved, cored, and sliced

2 tablespoons thinly sliced fresh sage leaves

½ cup low-sodium chicken broth

1 tablespoon whole-grain mustard

1. Heat the oil in a large nonstick skillet over medium-high heat. Dust the pork medallions on both sides with the pepper.

2. Cook the medallions in the hot pan, turning once, until browned and cooked through, about 4 minutes on each side. Transfer the medallions to a plate and tent them loosely with aluminum foil.

3. Reduce the heat to medium, add the shallots to the skillet, cover, and cook until the shallots are softened, about 5 minutes.

4. Add the vinegar and deglaze the pan, stirring to scrape up the browned bits from the bottom. Transfer the shallots to a small bowl.

5. Raise the heat to medium-high and add the butter, apple slices, and sage. Cook, stirring frequently, until the apples turn golden brown, 3 to 4 minutes.

6. Add the broth and mustard and stir to mix well. Simmer until the apples are quite soft, about 2 minutes more.

7. Return the shallots to the skillet and simmer until the sauce thickens, about 2 minutes.

8. Return the pork to the pan and cook, stirring, until heated through.

9. Serve the medallions topped with the apples, shallots, and sauce.

Grilled Steak Tacos with Fresh Salsa

SERVES 4

▶ *SODIUM //* **119 MG**
LOW-FAT // QUICK

When you hear the words "taco" and "steak," "healthful" and "low-fat" are probably not the first things that come to mind, but these grilled steak tacos are both low in fat and good for you. You'll get lots of iron and protein from the steak, and the salsa, cabbage, and radishes take care of your vegetable needs. You can substitute boneless, skinless chicken breast for the steak for an even lower-fat meal.

....

For the steak:
1 tablespoon chili powder
1 teaspoon brown sugar
1 teaspoon ground cumin
1 teaspoon dried oregano
½ teaspoon freshly ground pepper
⅛ teaspoon ground cinnamon
1 (1-pound) flank steak, trimmed

For the salsa:
2 large tomatoes, diced
1 small red onion, finely diced
¼ cup chopped fresh cilantro
1 jalapeño or serrano chili, seeded and finely diced
1 teaspoon lime zest
2 tablespoons fresh lime juice

For the tacos:
8 (6-inch) corn tortillas
2 cups shredded green cabbage
4 radishes, thinly sliced
Lime wedges, for garnish

....

To make the steak:

1. Preheat a barbecue or grill to medium-high heat.

2. In a bowl, combine the chili powder, sugar, cumin, oregano, pepper, and cinnamon. Rub the spice mixture over the steak.

3. Grill the steak, turning once, until the desired degree of doneness has been achieved, about 8 minutes per side for medium rare.

4. Transfer the steak to a cutting board, tent it loosely with foil, and let it rest for 10 minutes.

To make the salsa:

1. In a medium bowl, combine all the salsa ingredients and mix well. Let the salsa stand for 15 minutes or so before serving.

To make the tacos:

1. Preheat the oven to 350°F.

2. Wrap the tortillas in aluminum foil. Heat the tortillas in the oven for about 15 minutes.

3. When the steak has rested, cut it into ¼-inch-thick slices, cutting across the grain.

4. Place two warm tortillas on each serving plate. Divide the steak slices evenly among the tortillas and top each tortilla with ¼ cup of salsa and ¼ cup of cabbage. Tuck a few radish slices into each taco.

5. Serve the tacos with lime wedges on the side.

Grilled Steak with Arugula and Lemon Vinaigrette

SERVES 4

▶ *SODIUM //* **674 MG**

QUICK

Flat iron steak is a super-tender and flavorful cut that comes from the top part of the chuck roast. If you can't find flat iron steak, you can substitute New York strip steak, top sirloin steak, or even flank steak.

....

For the steak:

¾ cup chopped fresh flat-leaf parsley

2 tablespoons fresh lemon juice

1 tablespoon minced fresh oregano

2 garlic cloves, minced

1 tablespoon olive oil

½ teaspoon freshly ground pepper

2 boneless flat iron steaks, about 1½ inches thick

Cooking spray

For the vinaigrette:

1 teaspoon lemon zest

2 tablespoons fresh lemon juice

1 tablespoon white-wine vinegar or champagne vinegar

½ teaspoon Dijon mustard

½ teaspoon freshly ground pepper

Pinch of sugar

6 tablespoons olive oil

For serving:

2 (5-ounce) bags baby arugula

1 cup (about 4 ounces) shaved Parmesan cheese

....

To make the steak:

1. In a large bowl, whisk together the parsley, lemon juice, oregano, garlic, oil, and pepper. Add the steaks to the bowl and turn to coat. Cover and refrigerate the steak for 30 minutes.

2. Heat a grill, barbecue, or grill pan to medium-high heat and spray it with cooking spray.

3. Remove the steaks from the marinade, allowing any excess to drip off. Discard the marinade. Grill the steaks, turning once, until cooked to desired doneness, 3 to 4 minutes per side for medium rare.

4. Transfer the steak to a cutting board, tent it loosely with foil, and let it rest for 5 minutes.

5. Cut the steaks into ¼-inch-thick slices, cutting at an angle across the grain.

To make the vinaigrette:

1. In a small bowl, whisk together the lemon zest, lemon juice, vinegar, mustard, pepper, and sugar. Add the oil in a thin stream while whisking continuously until emulsified.

To serve:

1. Place the arugula in a large bowl. Add the vinaigrette and toss to coat well.

2. Arrange the dressed arugula on 4 serving plates, dividing it equally. Top the greens with the strips of steak, dividing it equally. Top the steak with the cheese, and serve immediately.

Nonna's Spaghetti and Meatballs

SERVES 4

▶ *SODIUM //* **218 MG**

LOW-FAT // MAKE AHEAD

If you don't have your own Italian grandmother, this recipe will ensure that you eat like you do. The meat is lightened up with brown rice (which keeps the recipe gluten-free, too) and moistened with minced mushrooms. While it takes a while to make, most of the time is hands-free. The prep is a cinch.

....

For the meatballs:

Olive oil cooking spray

1 pound lean ground beef

8 ounces cremini or button mushrooms, finely minced

½ cup uncooked brown rice

1 small onion, diced

¼ cup milk

1 egg

1 tablespoon fresh parsley, minced

1 teaspoon dried oregano

1 teaspoon garlic powder

½ teaspoon freshly ground pepper

¼ cup grated Parmesan cheese

For the sauce:

1 tablespoon olive oil

1 medium onion, diced

2 garlic cloves, minced

1 (28-ounce) can no-salt-added diced tomatoes, with juice

2 (14-ounce) cans no-salt-added tomato puree

1 (6-ounce) can tomato paste

1 teaspoon sugar

¾ teaspoon dried oregano

½ teaspoon freshly ground pepper

1 bay leaf

For serving:

1 pound dried spaghetti, cooked according to package directions

Grated Parmesan cheese, for serving (optional)

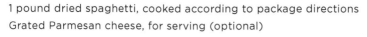

To make the meatballs:

1. Preheat the oven to 425°F.

2. Spray a large baking sheet with olive oil cooking spray.

3. In a large bowl, combine the beef, mushrooms, rice, onion, milk, egg, parsley, oregano, garlic powder, pepper, and cheese. Mix well, but do not overwork the mixture.

4. Shape the meat mixture into 1-inch meatballs and place them on the prepared baking sheet. Spritz the meatballs with the cooking spray and bake them in the oven for about 15 minutes to brown them.

To make the sauce:

1. Heat the oil in a large saucepan over medium heat. Add the onion and garlic and cook, stirring frequently, until the onion is softened, about 5 minutes.

2. Stir in the tomatoes with their juice, tomato puree, tomato paste, sugar, oregano, pepper, and bay leaf. Bring to a boil and then reduce the heat to medium-low.

3. Add the meatballs to the sauce and simmer, uncovered, stirring occasionally, for 2 to 3 hours.

To serve:

1. Spoon the cooked spaghetti into 4 bowls and pour the sauce and meatballs over it, dividing them equally. Offer additional Parmesan cheese for garnish, if desired.

CHAPTER FOURTEEN

Desserts

Desserts don't typically contain a lot of sodium, but they do often pack plenty of saturated fat and sugar. For those on a restricted diet, finding desserts that are healthful, low in fat and calories, and not too loaded with sugar, yet still satisfy a killer sweet tooth can be a challenge.

The recipes in this chapter focus on using healthful but super-flavorful ingredients like luscious berries and stone fruits, nutty coconut, dark chocolate, and brown sugar to pack a whole lot of deliciousness into these sweet delights. You'll find recipes for everything from quick treats to satisfy a sudden craving to elegant desserts worthy of your next dinner party.

Creamy Buttermilk-Lemon Sorbet

SERVES 4

▸ *SODIUM //* **132 MG**
LOW-FAT // MAKE AHEAD

Tangy and naturally low-fat buttermilk adds a creamy texture to this tart sorbet. Serve it topped with fresh blueberries or sliced fresh strawberries for a refreshing and satisfying summer dessert.

....

2 cups low-fat buttermilk
1 cup sugar
Zest of 1 lemon
¼ cup fresh lemon juice

....

1. In a large mixing bowl, stir all of the ingredients together until the sugar is completely dissolved.

2. Cover and refrigerate the mixture for about 4 hours, until it is very cold.

3. Transfer the mixture to an ice cream maker and freeze according to the manufacturer's instructions.

4. Transfer the sorbet to a freezer-safe container and freeze for at least 4 hours before serving.

Brown Sugar-Pecan Ice Cream

SERVES 8

▶ *SODIUM //* **89 MG**

LOW-FAT // MAKE AHEAD

Rich brown sugar flavor and toasty, nutty pecans come together in this low-fat ice cream, creating a delicious treat that won't derail your diet. Homemade ice cream is a cinch to make with an inexpensive ice cream maker.

1 tablespoon water

1½ teaspoons unflavored powdered gelatin

2½ cups low-fat milk

¾ cup packed dark brown sugar

½ teaspoon ground cinnamon

3 egg yolks

1 (12-ounce) can nonfat evaporated milk

1 teaspoon vanilla extract

½ cup chopped pecans

1. Place the water in a small bowl and sprinkle the gelatin over the top. Stir and then let sit for 10 minutes.

2. In a large saucepan, heat 1½ cups of the milk over medium heat. When the milk is hot, stir in the brown sugar and cinnamon, and continue to heat, whisking constantly, until the mixture is very hot but not boiling.

3. In a medium bowl, whisk together the egg yolks and evaporated milk.

4. Add the hot milk mixture to the egg mixture in a thin stream, whisking constantly, until well combined.

5. Transfer the mixture back to the saucepan and heat over medium heat, stirring constantly, until the mixture just begins to thicken, about 5 minutes. Be careful not to boil the mixture and curdle the eggs.

continued ▶

6. Strain the mixture through a fine-mesh sieve into a bowl and whisk in the gelatin and water mixture.

7. Stir in the remaining 1 cup of milk and the vanilla extract, cover, and chill in the refrigerator for at least 2 hours or overnight.

8. Stir the mixture, transfer it to an ice cream maker, and freeze it according to the manufacturer's instructions. When the mixture is almost frozen, add the pecans.

9. Transfer the ice cream to a freezer-safe container and freeze until firm. Serve frozen.

Ruby-Red Poached Pears

SERVES 4

▸ *SODIUM //* **8 MG**
LOW-FAT // MAKE AHEAD

Fresh pears take on a stunning ruby-red hue when they are poached in red wine. This luscious low-calorie dessert is practically fat-free, but its gorgeous appearance makes it a suitable end to an elegant dinner party. Serve it with vanilla ice cream or frozen yogurt, if desired.

2 cups red wine
¼ cup sugar
1 (3-inch) strip of orange peel
Juice of 1 orange
1 cinnamon stick
2 whole cloves
4 firm, ripe pears, peeled, stems left intact, and bottoms
    leveled so the pears will stand up

1. In a large saucepan, bring the wine, sugar, orange peel, orange juice, cinnamon stick, and cloves to a boil over medium-high heat. Reduce the heat to medium-low and simmer, uncovered, for about 5 minutes.

2. Add the pears to the liquid, cover, and cook, turning the pears occasionally, for about 20 minutes, until the pears are tender but not soft. Transfer the pears to a platter or large bowl.

3. Raise the heat to medium-high and cook the liquids, stirring, for about 15 minutes, until the mixture begins to thicken and get syrupy.

4. Remove the orange peel, cinnamon stick, and cloves.

5. Pour the sauce over the pears and chill for 2 hours or more before serving.

Peach-Blueberry Crisp with Coconut Topping

SERVES 4

▶ *SODIUM //* **6 MG**
LOW-FAT

Crisps are a favorite dessert option in the summer when stone fruits and berries are at their peak. This recipe combines the two for a pretty crisp that is light and delicious. In the fall, you might substitute apples or pears and cranberries. A double dose of coconut makes this version unique and especially nutritious. Cooking and serving it in individual ramekins makes both portion control and cleaning up a snap.

For the filling:
Cooking spray
2 cups sliced peaches
1 cup fresh blueberries
2 tablespoons granulated sugar
2 tablespoons all-purpose flour
2 tablespoons fresh lemon juice

For the topping:
¾ cup old-fashioned rolled oats
¼ cup all-purpose flour
3 tablespoons unsweetened coconut flakes
2 tablespoons coconut oil
¼ cup packed brown sugar

To make the filling:

1. Preheat the oven to 350°F.

2. Spray four 8-ounce ramekins lightly with cooking spray. Set the ramekins on a baking sheet.

3. In a large bowl, toss together the peaches and blueberries. Add the sugar, flour, and lemon juice and toss to combine.

4. Spoon the mixture into the prepared ramekins, dividing it equally.

To make the topping:

1. Combine the oats, flour, coconut flakes, coconut oil, and brown sugar in a food processor. Pulse until the mixture is well combined.

2. Spoon the mixture over the fruit in the ramekins, dividing it equally and making sure to cover the fruit completely.

3. Place the baking sheet with the filled ramekins on it in the oven and bake for about 1 hour, until the top is nicely browned and the filling is very hot and bubbling.

4. Serve warm, topped with a scoop of vanilla ice cream or frozen yogurt, if desired.

Sour Cream and Cinnamon Coffee Cake

SERVES 10

▶ *SODIUM //* **85 MG**
LOW-FAT

This classic coffee cake recipe with a crumbly cinnamon topping is a fantastic light dessert, and the leftovers make a lovely breakfast the next morning.

....

For the topping:
½ cup sugar
½ cup all-purpose flour
1 teaspoon ground cinnamon
2 tablespoons unsalted butter, melted

For the cake:
Cooking spray
All-purpose flour, for dusting
1⅓ cups cake flour
1 teaspoon baking powder
⅛ teaspoon baking soda
¼ cup (½ stick) unsalted butter, at room temperature
¼ cup low-fat plain yogurt
¾ cup sugar
1 egg yolk
1 egg, at room temperature
½ cup reduced-fat sour cream, at room temperature
1 teaspoon vanilla extract

....

To make the topping:

1. In a medium mixing bowl, combine the sugar, flour, and cinnamon.

2. Stir in the melted butter until well combined.

To make the cake:

1. Preheat the oven to 350°F.

2. Spray an 8 by 8-inch square or 9-inch round baking pan with cooking spray, and dust lightly with flour.

3. In a small mixing bowl, combine the cake flour, baking powder, and baking soda.

4. In a large mixing bowl, stir together the butter, yogurt, sugar, and egg yolk until well combined.

5. Add the egg and whisk until the mixture is smooth.

6. Add the sour cream and vanilla and stir to combine.

7. Add the dry ingredients to the wet ingredients and whisk until smooth.

8. Transfer the batter to the prepared baking pan. Top the batter with the topping mixture and spread out to an even layer.

9. Bake the cake for 25 to 30 minutes, until the topping is golden brown and a toothpick inserted into the center of the cake comes out clean.

10. Cool the cake in the pan on a wire rack for 10 to 15 minutes before serving. Serve warm.

Lemon Meringue Layer Cake

SERVES 12

▶ *SODIUM //* **79 MG**
LOW-FAT

*Fresh lemon juice and lemon zest make this beautiful and light layer cake a
tantalizing tart. The creamy but light meringue provides a stunning topping,
making this cake perfect for a special occasion.*

....

For the cake:
Cooking spray
All-purpose flour, for dusting
4 eggs, at room temperature
⅔ cup sugar
1 teaspoon vanilla extract
1 teaspoon lemon zest
3 tablespoons canola oil
¾ cup cake flour

For the filling:
1 (14-ounce) can fat-free sweetened condensed milk
1 teaspoon lemon zest
⅓ cup fresh lemon juice

For the topping:
2 egg whites, at room temperature
¼ teaspoon cream of tartar
¼ cup sugar
¼ teaspoon vanilla extract

....

To make the cake:

1. Preheat the oven to 350°F.

2. Spray two 9-inch round cake pans with cooking spray and then dust with flour.

3. In a large bowl, combine the eggs and sugar and beat with an electric mixer set on medium-high speed until fluffy and pale yellow, 8 to 10 minutes. Add the vanilla and lemon zest.

4. Using a rubber spatula, gently fold in the oil.

5. Stir in the flour just until incorporated.

6. Transfer the batter to the prepared baking pans, dividing it evenly.

7. Bake the cakes for 20 to 22 minutes, until a toothpick inserted into the center comes out clean.

8. Place the pans on a wire rack to cool for 10 minutes, then turn the cakes out onto the rack and cool completely.

To make the filling:

1. In a medium bowl, stir together the condensed milk, lemon zest, and lemon juice until well combined.

2. Chill for 30 minutes (or as long as overnight).

To make the topping:

1. Place the egg whites and cream of tartar in a medium mixing bowl and whip with an electric mixer set on high until soft peaks form.

2. While continuing to whip the mixture, add the sugar 1 tablespoon at a time.

3. Add the vanilla extract.

4. Whip until stiff peaks form.

5. Preheat the broiler.

6. To assemble the cake, first place one of the cake layers, convex side up, on a baking sheet. Spread the topping decoratively over the cake layer with a spatula or pipe it using a pastry bag.

7. Place the cake under the broiler and broil just until the topping is golden brown, about 1 minute. Remove the cake from the broiler.

8. Set the other cake layer, flat side up, on a cake plate and spread the filling over the top evenly. Place the layer with the topping on top.

9. Cut the cake into wedges and serve.

Light and Luscious Chocolate Cream Pie

SERVES 8

▸ *SODIUM //* **116 MG**
LOW-FAT // MAKE AHEAD

Thought you had to give up indulgent treats like chocolate cream pie? Think again. This lightened-up version is low in fat but doesn't skimp on the rich chocolate flavor. Serve it topped with fresh fruit or whipped topping for a special dessert.

For the crust:
1¼ cups (about 30 wafers) chocolate cookie crumbs, such as Famous Wafers
3 tablespoons unsalted butter, melted

For the filling:
¾ cup sugar
¼ cup cornstarch
¼ cup unsweetened cocoa powder
1¾ cups low-fat milk or light coconut milk
1 egg
4 ounces bittersweet chocolate, finely chopped
Fresh raspberries, sliced strawberries, or sliced bananas, for serving (optional)
Fat-free nondairy whipped topping, for serving (optional)

To make the crust:

1. Process the cookies in a food processor until finely ground.

2. Add the butter and process until the crumbs are thoroughly moistened.

3. Press the crumbs into the bottom and up the sides of a 9-inch pie plate.

4. Chill until firm.

To make the filling:

1. In a large saucepan set over medium heat, whisk together the sugar, cornstarch, and cocoa. Add the milk and egg and continue whisking until smooth.

2. Cook, stirring constantly, until the mixture bubbles and thickens, about 5 minutes.

3. Remove the mixture from the heat and add the chocolate, stirring until it is fully melted and incorporated.

4. Pour the filling into the prepared crust, cover with plastic wrap, pressing the plastic onto the surface of the filling, and chill until set, at least 4 hours.

5. Serve chilled, topped with fruit or whipped topping, if desired.

No-Bake Chocolate-Glazed Coconut Bars

MAKES 8 BARS

▶ *SODIUM //* **4 MG** *(PER BAR)*
LOW-FAT // QUICK

Besides being unbelievably delicious, coconut provides your body with medium-chain fatty acids, which help lower cholesterol. These quick and easy-to-make bars contain a triple dose of coconut (meat, cream, and oil), with delicious and good-for-you dark chocolate. It's healthful food that tastes like candy.

....

For the bars:
1½ cups shredded unsweetened coconut
¼ cup sugar
2 tablespoons coconut cream
2 tablespoons coconut oil
½ teaspoon vanilla extract

For the chocolate glaze:
3 tablespoons mini dark chocolate chips
½ tablespoon coconut oil

....

To make the bars:

1. In a medium bowl, stir together the shredded coconut, sugar, coconut cream, coconut oil, and vanilla until well combined.

2. Press the mixture into an 8 by 8-inch baking pan.

3. Chill the bars in the freezer for 15 minutes, until firm.

4. Line a baking sheet with parchment paper.

To make the chocolate glaze:

1. In a microwave-safe glass measuring cup with a spout or a small microwave-safe bowl, combine the chocolate chips and the coconut oil. Heat the chocolate and oil in a microwave on 50 percent power for 30 seconds at a time until the chocolate chips are halfway melted.

3. Stir to melt them completely and combine the mixture well.

4. Remove the bars from the freezer and cut into 8 bars. Place the bars on the prepared baking sheet and drizzle the chocolate glaze over the top.

5. Place the baking sheet in the freezer for another 5 minutes or so, until the chocolate has set.

6. Serve immediately or store the bars in the refrigerator for up to 3 weeks.

Cherry-Almond Biscotti

MAKES 18 BISCOTTI

▶ *SODIUM //* **63 MG** *(PER BISCOTTI)*
LOW-FAT

Biscotti are the perfect sweet—but not too sweet—treat to go with a cup of coffee after a meal or anytime you need a treat. Tart dried cherries are loaded with disease-fighting antioxidants. The fact that they may help to prevent insomnia—they contain the hormone melatonin, which helps regulate sleep cycles—make these low-fat biscuits an ideal after-dinner snack. Of course, you'll want to pair them with a cup of (decaffeinated) coffee for dunking.

....

1 cup all-purpose flour
1 cup whole-wheat flour
½ teaspoon baking powder
½ teaspoon baking soda
¼ cup (½ stick) unsalted butter, at room temperature
½ cup granulated sugar
¼ cup brown sugar
2 eggs
1 tablespoon vanilla extract
3 ounces almonds
2 ounces dried cherries, chopped

....

1. Preheat the oven to 350°F.

2. Line a baking sheet with parchment paper.

3. In a medium mixing bowl, stir together the flours, baking powder, and baking soda.

4. In a large mixing bowl, using an electric mixer, beat the butter and the sugars together until creamy.

5. Add the eggs, one at a time, beating after each addition until just incorporated.

6. Add the vanilla and the dry ingredients and beat until well combined. Add the almonds and the dried cherries.

7. Split the dough into 2 equal portions. On the prepared baking sheet, shape the dough into two 3 by 8-inch loaves.

8. Bake the loaves until they are golden, 30 to 35 minutes.

9. Remove the baking sheet from the oven, reduce the oven heat to 325°F, and let the loaves cool for 15 minutes or so.

10. Cut the loaves at a 45-degree angle into 1-inch-wide slices.

11. Return the slices to the baking sheet, standing them on their uncut edges. Bake the biscotti until they are very dry and lightly browned, about 25 minutes.

12. Cool completely on a wire rack and serve at room temperature.

The Best Oatmeal-Chocolate Chip Cookies

MAKES ABOUT 30 COOKIES (1 COOKIE PER SERVING)

▶ *SODIUM //* **17 MG** *(PER COOKIE)*
LOW-FAT

There's nothing quite as nice as the smell of homemade cookies baking in the oven, except perhaps that first ooey, gooey, fresh-out-of-the-oven bite. This lightened-up version of the classic cookie won't disappoint. They are full of chewy oats, luscious dark chocolate, and the caramel sweetness of brown sugar.

....

½ cup all-purpose flour
½ cup whole-wheat flour
¾ cup old-fashioned quick-cooking rolled oats
½ teaspoon baking powder
⅓ teaspoon baking soda
¾ cup light brown sugar
⅓ cup canola oil
1 egg
1 teaspoon vanilla extract
⅓ cup dark chocolate chips

....

1. Preheat the oven to 350°F.

2. Line a large baking sheet with parchment paper.

3. In a medium mixing bowl, combine the flours, oats, baking powder, and baking soda.

4. Using an electric mixer, in a large mixing bowl, cream together the sugar and oil.

5. Add the egg and vanilla and beat to combine.

6. Add the dry mixture to the wet mixture and beat to combine.

7. Fold in the chocolate chips.

8. Drop the cookie dough onto the baking sheet by rounded tablespoons.

9. Bake the cookies until golden brown, about 25 minutes. Transfer the cookies to a wire rack to cool.

10. Serve warm or at room temperature.

Appendix A:
Shopping Tips

Low-Sodium Diet Shopping Tips

Shopping for low-sodium food will be a learning experience in the beginning, and you may need to allow extra time to do your grocery shopping at first as you'll be spending time reading labels and comparing brands. Once you find products you like and that fit into your new diet, you'll be able to get your groceries just as quickly as ever. Consider these useful tips to help make your grocery shopping easier and more nutritious.

Shop Around the Edges of the Store

Buy the majority of your foods from the fresh food sections, which are normally located around the edges of the store. This includes fresh fruits and vegetables, fresh meats, seafood, poultry, and fresh dairy products. Load up your cart with these items and you'll be well on your way to a low-sodium meal plan.

Skip the Danger Zones

Stay out of the aisles where processed snacks, such as chips and cookies, are located. Out of sight, out of mind. When you do venture into the inner aisles of the store, be sure you've got your reading glasses handy. You'll need to read every label, checking the sodium content as well as the serving size so that you know how much sodium you'll be getting for the quantity you are likely to eat in a meal.

Read Your Labels

Don't assume that something is low in sodium just because it isn't salty. Read the labels on everything. It's always best to make your food from scratch so that you can control the sodium content, but that isn't possible for everyone. When you need to buy prepared foods, buy those that are lowest in sodium, sugar, and saturated fat. Make note of the best brands so you can eventually shop without having to do any heavy reading. Don't just stop at reading one label for a given food. Compare brands and you might find that the same food from one brand is much lower or higher in sodium than from another. And remember, it's not just canned, jarred, and snack foods whose labels you need to read. Check each and every food that has a label—including dairy products, breakfast cereals, and grains.

Buy the Rainbow

To ensure a high intake of antioxidants and micronutrients, choose different kinds of produce every time you shop. Don't just buy green peppers—buy red or orange peppers. Choose lots of dark, leafy greens. Buy fruits that are rich in color, such as watermelon, mango, and dark berries. Consuming a diverse variety of produce will help increase each bite's nutritional value.

Choose Your Meat and Seafood Wisely

Whenever possible, buy organic, grass-fed, or pasture-raised meats and wild seafood; they have more omega-3 fatty acids and are more likely to be free of hormones and preservatives. Always choose the leanest cuts of whatever you're buying, and trim visible fat after cooking.

Choose Low-Fat Dairy

Low-fat dairy products should be chosen whenever possible. Cheeses should be nonfat or partially nonfat. Milk should be nonfat or one percent fat. Yogurt should be nonfat and low in sugar or sugar-free.

Appendix B

Resources

Diets are most successful when you arm yourself with the right tools. The following websites provide a wealth of information and resources to help you find success with your low-sodium diet.

Online Stores

Healthy Heart Market

This online retailer carries low-sodium, sodium-free, and no-salt-added foods. Here you'll find everything from low-sodium baking essentials to spices and seasoning mixes, condiments, sauces, soups, salsas, salad dressings, pickles, snacks, and more.
www.healthyheartmarket.com
(800)-753-0310

Informational Websites

The American Heart Association

The American Heart Association's website provides extensive information about heart disease, stroke, high blood pressure, and other conditions, including symptoms, risk factors, preventive measures, and treatment information.
www.heart.org

DASH Diet

This website provides information about Dietary Alternatives to Stop Hypertension (DASH) and the DASH Diet Eating Plan. The DASH Diet was developed as a way to lower high blood pressure without medication. This website provides information on the background of the diet, diet tips, and recipes.
www.dashdiet.org

Heart Healthy Online

This website offers extensive information about heart disease, stroke, blood pressure, and cholesterol, including how to recognize symptoms of disease, how to get help, and tips on how to reduce your risk. It also offers heart healthful recipes, fitness advice, and information on stress management.
www.hearthealthyonline.com

The Mayo Clinic

The Mayo Clinic's website includes information on the symptoms, causes, and treatments of high blood pressure, including medications and dietary and lifestyle changes.
www.mayoclinic.com

National Heart, Lung, and Blood Institute

This website provides information on high blood pressure as well as advice for lowering blood pressure through diet and exercise.
www.nhlbi.nih.gov

WebMD

At the WebMD site, you'll find information, supportive community forums, and in-depth reference material about a vast range of health topics, including hypertension, stroke, heart disease, kidney disease, and more. They also provide information on how to follow a low-sodium diet, including meal plans and recipes.
www.webmd.com

Dr. Weil

This website provides extensive information on dietary and lifestyle changes that may significantly reduce blood pressure and the risk of heart disease, stroke, and other diseases.
www.drweil.com

References

Esselstyn, Caldwell B., Jr. *Prevent and Reverse Heart Disease: The Revolutionary, Scientifically Proven, Nutrition-Based Cure*. New York: Avery, 2007.

Gillinov, Marc, and Steven Nissen. *Heart 411: The Only Guide to Heart Health You'll Ever Need*. New York: Three Rivers Press, 2012.

Heller, Marla. *The DASH Diet Action Plan: Proven to Boost Weight Loss and Improve Health*. Northbrook, IL: Amidon Press, 2007.

Kowalski, Robert E. *The Blood Pressure Cure: 8 Weeks to Lower Blood Pressure without Prescription Drugs*. New Jersey: Wiley, 2007.

Mateljan, George. *The World's Healthiest Foods: Essential Guide for the Healthiest Way of Eating*. Seattle: George Mateljan Foundation, 2005.

Moore, Thomas, Laura Svetkey, Pao-Hwa Lin, Njeri Karanja, and Mark Jenkins. *The DASH Diet for Hypertension: Lower Your Blood Pressure in 14 Days—without Drugs*. New York: Pocket Books, 2003.

Nestle, Marion. *What to Eat*. New York: North Point Press, 2006.

Index

Printed in Great Britain
by Amazon.co.uk, Ltd.,
Marston Gate.